AEROBIC

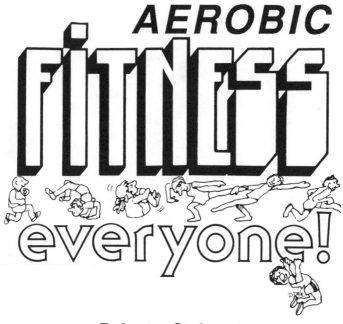

FITNESS
everyone!

Roberta Stokes
Diane E. Trapp

Miami-Dade Community College
Miami, Florida

▟▙ Hunter Textbooks Inc.

ISBN 0-88725-114-5

Inquiries should be addressed to the publisher:

⊞ Hunter Textbooks Inc.

823 Reynolda Road
Winston-Salem, North Carolina 27104

PREFACE

Interest in health and personal fitness is rapidly increasing among all Americans. People are recognizing the importance of achieving optimal levels of fitness rather than being satisfied with just average. In attempting to reshape and change their bodies, more Americans increasingly are setting personal goals and accepting the responsibility for making changes in their lifestyle.

Why *aerobic* fitness? The major goal of this text is to assist you in achieving your optimal level of aerobic fitness. The special emphasis on aerobic fitness is because of its important role in overall health and wellness. A sound program of exercise which leads to aerobic fitness also contributes significantly to a program of weight control, and can play a major role in managing stress. The most important muscle you have is your heart, and by achieving an optimal level of aerobic fitness, you are improving the functioning of this vital organ. Of course, balance in life is also essential. Therefore, you will find additional resources on the other aspects necessary for total fitness: flexibility, muscular strength and endurance, nutrition, weight control, and stress management.

Our major objective is to challenge each reader to reach high — to seek the greatest possible level of health and fitness. Is your current lifestyle worth dying for? Why not make the commitment to change today? The choice is yours!

CONTENTS

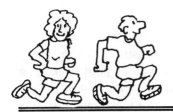

Chapter One

Seeing the Whole Picture
OPTIMAL FITNESS

The word *fitness* means different things to different people. There are various levels of fitness and various components of fitness. Optimal fitness refers to one's highest possible level of overall health. Unfortunately, the average person does not live at an optimal level of health or fitness. Most seem satisfied to reach minimal standards rather than attaining the highest attainable level of health — optimal fitness. Our error in the past has been in believing that reaching a "normal" or average level implied we were in good health. We now know that such standards are misleading because our population has a high incidence of obesity, hypertension, smoking; a poor level of physical fitness; and a diet high in calories, fat, and cholesterol. Therefore, only by seeking optimal standards can we be assured of the highest level of health.

The key to attaining an optimal level of health and fitness is a change in lifestyle. There is little doubt that today's lifestyle contributes to our being unfit but this can be changed. We can make different choices regarding exercise, smoking, diet, and managing stress, but we need to initiate these changes as early as possible. The evidence is clear that we can affect our chances of living longer at almost any time in our lives, but the earlier we start the greater the effect will be.

How can we achieve optimal fitness? First, we must analyze our behavior and lifestyle to determine what changes need to be made. Second, we need to evaluate our current fitness level to identify strengths and weaknesses; and third, we must establish goals for improvement, then plan and follow an individualized training program.

LIFESTYLE CHANGES

Three important areas of lifestyle should be examined for possible change: activity, diet, and stress.

In today's sedentary society our daily tasks of living no longer require rigorous physical activity. In addition, most of us usually look for every possible way of avoiding exercise — we ride rather than walk, use elevators instead of stairs, sit and watch television rather than be active, and use every labor-saving device possible. We simply must turn this around so that activity becomes a regular part of our lives. Exercise can be planned to fit any busy schedule and become a daily habit.

Our daily nutritional habits also need review. We can bring our intake of nutrients in line with those recommended for optimal nutrition. We can eliminate or decrease excessive calories, fat, cholesterol, sugar, and salt from our diet. Dietary habits are not easy to change but the choice is yours.

Another area of lifestyle which must be examined is the control of stress. The increased pressures brought about by the complexities of modern civilization are taking a tremendous toll on most Americans. The stress of our lifestyles contributes to and is associated with numerous psychological and even physical disorders. We must become more aware of stress factors and learn how to cope with them. Effective techniques can be employed if the problem is first identified.

If your motivation is strong enough, you can make the changes in your lifestyle that will help you achieve optimal fitness.

Three areas of your lifestyle to examine for change:
ACTIVITY
DIET
STRESS

FITNESS EVALUATION

Numerous tests have indicated the general lack of minimal levels of physical fitness among American children and adults. As a nation we have not recognized the necessity of regular exercise for our personal health and well-being. Regardless of age, we now must take the time to learn how to evaluate individual strengths and weaknesses. We need to know which specific areas of our personal fitness need improvement and then we can set realistic goals for change. There are four major components of physical fitness relating directly to a person's health: cardiovascular endurance, flexibility, muscular strength and endurance, and body composition.

Cardiovascular endurance is the most important element of physical fitness. It is a measure of the ability of the heart, lungs, and blood vessels to function effectively. A high level of cardiovascular endurance is essential, not only to achieving fitness but to the performance of our everyday activities. The main theme of this book, aerobic fitness, relates to attaining a high level of cardiovascular endurance.

Flexibility is the capacity of a joint to move through its entire range of motion. Lack of flexibility may result in postural problems, muscle injury and soreness, limitation of movement, inability to perform daily tasks, and restricted performance of many sport skills. Studies show that the most frequent cause of loss of flexibility is lack of continued exercise.

Body Composition refers to the percentage of body weight that is fat in relation to that which is lean muscle mass. Excessive accumulation of body fat (obesity) is closely related to many physical and emotional problems. If you are to reach your state of optimal fitness, body weight and percentage of fat must be kept within an acceptable range.

Muscular strength and endurance are important components of physical fitness and are closely related. Strength refers to the ability of a muscle to exert force against resistance. Muscular endurance is the ability of a muscle to exert force continuously over a period of time. Therefore, if a muscle grows stronger its ability to continue to contract without fatigue will be greater. Increased muscular endurance will enable you to perform simple household tasks more effectively and improve your sports performance. In addition, muscles that are stronger will be less susceptible to injury from strains and sprains. Since fitness is constantly changing one, we must periodically reassess our status. That is one of the challenges that achieving fitness presents — **we must make a lifelong commitment to it.**

THE TRAINING PROGRAM

Perhaps the key to obtaining optimal fitness is the establishment of specific goals and the commitment to an individualized training program. You must develop a positive plan for changing your lifestyle in all areas and actually participate in a regular exercise program. Since exercise is an individual matter, a variety of training programs can be followed. What is important is that you find an activity that is right for you—one that meets your needs and interests, one you can stay with throughout your life. Of course, exercise alone cannot do it all, but certainly it is a proven method for attaining a high level of fitness.

There is no doubt that a commitment to change your lifestyle will require time, effort, and sacrifice. Along the way you may experience discouragement, doubt, and failure. However, keeping in mind the benefits of reaching a goal of optimal fitness may help you to maintain your determination. Some of the specific outcomes of achieving optimal fitness and participating in a regular program of physical activity are listed in the box on the next page.

Physiological Benefits of Exercise

1. Reduces the number of heartbeats per minute (heart rate) by increasing the amount of blood pumped per beat (stroke volume), thus improving the efficiency of the heart.
2. Lowers blood pressure by increasing the number of functional capillaries in the muscles.
3. Increases lean muscle tissue and decreases total body fat by utilizing fat as the major fuel source.
4. Increases high-density lipoproteins (good, protective cholesterol) levels in the blood, which reduces the risk of heart disease.
5. Improves muscular endurance and increases energy levels by enhancing the oxygen transport system.
6. Increases the effectiveness of weight-loss programs by elevating the metabolic rate during and after exercise.
7. Retards the aging process.

Psychological Benefits of Exercise

1. Enhances appearance and improves self-image, which promotes self-confidence and overall feeling of well-being.
2. Increases the ability to handle stress and decreases anxiety levels.
3. Makes work and leisure time activity more productive and meaningful.
4. Promotes relaxation and increases the ability to cope.
5. Enhances the effectiveness of sleep by decreasing the amount needed and increasing the quality.

Chapter Two will start you toward your goal by suggesting evaluation methods to assess your current level of fitness.

REFERENCES

1. Allsen, P., Harrison, J., and Vance, B. *Fitness for Life.* Wm. C. Brown Co. Dubuque, Iowa, 1984.
2. Cooper, Kenneth. *The Aerobics Program for a Total Well-Being.* M. Evans & Company, Inc., New York, 1982.
3. Falls, H., Baylor, A., and Dishman, R. *Essentials of Fitness.* Saunders, Philadelphia, 1980.
4. Garrison, L., Leslie, P., and Blackmore, D. *Fitness and Figure Control.* Mayfield Publishing Co., Palo Alto, California, 1981.
5. Getchell, Bud. *The Fitness Book.* Benchmark Press, Inc., Indianapolis, Indiana, 1987.
6. Getchell, Bud. *Physical Fitness: A Way of Life.* John Wiley & Sons, New York, 1983.
7. Golding, L., Myers, C., and Sinning, W. (eds). *The Y's Way to Physical Fitness.* National Board of YMCA, Chicago, 1982.
8. Hockey, Robert V. *Physical Fitness — The Pathway to Healthful Living.* C.V. Mosby Co., St. Louis, 1985.
9. Miller, David and Allen, T. Earl. *Fitness: A Lifetime Commitment.* Burgess Publishing Co., Minneapolis, 1986.
11. Stokes, R., Moore, A., Moore, C. *Fitness: The New Wave.* Hunter Textbooks Inc., Winston-Salem, NC, 1988.
10. U.S. Dept. of Health and Human Services. *Exercise and Your Heart.* U.S. Government Printing Office, 1981.

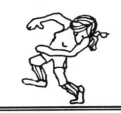

Chapter Two

Understanding the Problem
ASSESSMENT OF CURRENT FITNESS

How physically fit are you? Are you in good health? Have you had a physical examination recently? How active have you been? Can you perform daily activities without tiring easily? Do you have an acceptable level of body fat? These are important questions which need to be examined before beginning an exercise program.

Assessment of your current level of fitness should begin with a review of your family and personal health history. Lab 2 contains a sample health questionnaire. Its purpose is to detect disorders that might prevent or restrict your participation in a regular exercise program, and to evaluate your degree of heart attack risk. It is extremely important that all questions be answered as accurately as possible so that an effective and safe individual program may be developed. If there are any doubts about the advisability of your participation in an exercise program, you should first consult a physician.

The next step is to determine your current physical condition so that personal improvement goals and an appropriate training program can be designed. This can be accomplished by participating in a series of physical fitness tests. Since physical fitness has more than one dimension, several tests are needed to assess it. You may score well on some tests and not so well on others. Hopefully, the test results will motivate you to seek improvement and establish a regular exercise program. By repeating the tests periodically, you can evaluate your progress and determine the effectiveness of your training program.

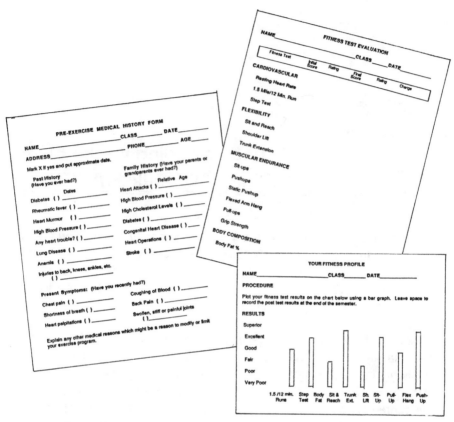

After completing the tests and activities described in this chapter, you will be able to establish your physical fitness profile and compare your results to others of your age and sex who have previously completed the tests. However, the establishment of precise test norms and standards is difficult and therefore norms should only be used as a guide to aid in assessing your particular strengths and weaknesses — not as a means of comparing yourself to others. Actually, you should concentrate on improving your scores and measure your own individual improvement. You should also establish a goal of optimal physical fitness for *you*. The optimal level refers to the achievement of your maximum potential. Each of us is unique and will improve at a different rate, so do not become discouraged if others seem to develop more quickly than you. Just strive to do the best you can and to continue to progress toward your goal.

8

EVALUATING CARDIOVASCULAR ENDURANCE

Cardiovascular endurance is a measure of the ability of the heart to pump blood, of the lungs to process volumes of air, and of the muscles to utilize oxygen. Tests designed to measure cardiovascular endurance involve vigorous physical activity that make high demands on the heart and lungs. One's level of cardiovascular endurance is generally considered the most important single measure of the overall level of fitness because it reflects the condition of the heart, blood vessels, and lungs, as well as the general condition of the muscles.

One-Mile Walking Test

For those individuals who are considerably overweight, who have been inactive for some time, or are over 35 years of age, it is recommended that a walking test be attempted before more strenuous cardiovascular tests. A simple, safe test which can be used to identify a general level of fitness is to walk a mile for time. This test involves finding an area which measures one mile and walking it as quickly as possible. The time it takes to complete the walk indicates the general fitness category as follows:

Time to Walk Mile	Fitness Category
<10 minutes	high
11-12 minutes	above average
12-15 minutes	average
15-20 minutes	below average
> 20 minutes	low

Depending on your test results and how you feel when you finish, you may find it necessary to begin a walking program before taking a running test.

Run-Walk Tests

12 Minute Run-Walk Test. One simple test for measuring cardiovascular endurance is the 12 minute run-walk test. This test has been found to give a reliable estimate of one's maximal oxygen consumption and can be used in place of more extensive tests such as the treadmill or bicycle ergometer test. The test involves measuring the distance covered by running, or running and walking, for 12 minutes. The purpose is to cover as much distance as possible; however, the test should not be continued if extreme fatigue, dizziness, shortness of breath, or nausea are experienced. Ratings of your cardiovascular endurance based on the 12 minute run-walk are given below.

12-MINUTE RUN-WALK RATINGS

RATING	FEMALES (BY AGE)					
	13-19	20-29	30-39	40-49	50-59	60 +
Superior	>1.52	>1.46	>1.40	>1.35	>1.31	>1.19
Excellent	1.44-1.51	1.35-1.45	1.30-1.39	1.25-1.34	1.19-1.30	1.10-1.18
Good	1.30-1.43	1.23-1.34	1.19-1.29	1.12-1.24	1.06-1.18	.99-1.09
Fair	1.19-1.29	1.12-1.22	1.06-1.18	.99-1.11	.94-1.05	.87-.98
Poor	1.00-1.18	.96-1.11	.95-1.05	.88-.98	.84-.93	.78-.86
Very Poor	<1.00	<.96	<.95	<.88	<.84	<.78

RATING	MALES (BY AGE)					
	13-19	20-29	30-39	40-49	50-59	60 +
Superior	>1.87	>1.77	>1.70	>1.66	>1.59	>1.56
Excellent	1.73-1.86	1.65-1.76	1.57-1.69	1.54-1.65	1.45-1.58	1.33-1.55
Good	1.57-1.72	1.50-1.64	1.46-1.56	1.40-1.53	1.31-1.44	1.21-1.32
Fair	1.38-1.56	1.32-1.49	1.31-1.45	1.25-1.39	1.17-1.30	1.03-1.20
Poor	1.30-1.37	1.22-1.31	1.18-1.30	1.14-1.24	1.03-1.16	.87-1.02
Very Poor	<1.30	<1.22	<1.18	<1.14	<1.03	<.87

1.5 Mile Run-Walk Test. An alternate test for determining cardiovascular endurance is the 1.5 mile run-walk test. The time it takes the individual to run-walk a distance of 1.5 miles is recorded to the nearest hundredth of a second. One should observe the same precautions as with the 12 minute run-walk test, but attempt to cover the distance in the shortest possible time.

Ratings of cardiovascular endurance based on the 1.5 mile run-walk are given below.

1.5 MILE RUN RATINGS

FITNESS CATEGORY	FEMALES (BY AGE)					
	13-19	20-29	30-39	40-49	50-59	60 -
Superior	<11:50	<12:30	<13:00	<13:45	<14:30	<16:30
Excellent	11:50-12:29	12:30-13:30	13:00-14:30	13:45-15:55	14:30-16:30	16:30-17:30
Good	12:30-14:30	13:31-15:54	14:31-16:30	15:56-17:30	16:31-19:00	17:31-19:30
Fair	14:31-16:54	15:55-18:30	16:31-19:00	17:31-19:30	19:01-20:00	19:31-20:30
Poor	16:55-18:30	18:31-19:00	19:01-19:30	19:31-20:00	20:01-20:30	20:31-21:00
Very Poor	>18:31	>19:01	>19:31	>20:01	>20:31	>21:01

FITNESS CATEGORY	MALES (BY AGE)					
	13-19	20-29	30-39	40-49	50-59	60 -
Superior	<8:37	<9:45	<10:00	<10:30	<11:00	<11:15
Excellent	8:37-9:40	9:45-10:45	10:00-11:00	10:30-11:30	11:00-12:30	11:15-13:59
Good	9:41-10:48	10:46-12:00	11:01-12:30	11:31-13:00	12:31-14:30	14:00-16:15
Fair	10:49-12:10	12:01-14:00	12:31-14:45	13:01-15:35	14:31-17:00	16:16-19:00
Poor	12:11-15:30	14:01-16:00	14:46-16:30	15:36-17:30	17:01-19:00	19:01-20:00
Very Poor	>15:31	>16:10	>16:31	>17:31	>19:01	>20:01

Resting Heart Rate

Another measure of cardiovascular efficiency is the resting heart rate. The best way to measure the resting heart rate is to take the pulse upon waking in the morning, and while still in bed. The resting pulse may also be measured by selecting a time when you have not done any physical activity for at least 30 minutes, have not eaten for several hours and feel relaxed. A lower resting heart rate is desired since it is an indication that the heart is working more efficiently in meeting the body's demand for blood. It also means a greater stroke volume, which indicates that more blood is pumped with each beat allowing the heart more time for rest between beats. Studies show that people who develop high levels of cardiovascular endurance often have resting rates below 50 beats per minute. The American Heart Association identifies the normal range for resting heart rates as being between 50-100 beats per minute. The resting heart rate will decrease gradually in response to a program of regular endurance activities. By keeping a record of your resting pulse rate, you can chart the progress you are making in your training program.

Counting Your Pulse

The pulse can be counted most accurately by applying light pressure to the radial artery on the inside of your wrist. Place the tips of the first two fingers on the wrist just below the base of the thumb and press lightly. When you feel the pulse, count the number of beats for the appropriate time period using a stop watch or a watch with a second hand. An alternate spot for finding the pulse is the carotid artery, which is found by placing two fingers lightly under the jawbone, slightly to the back of the Adam's Apple.

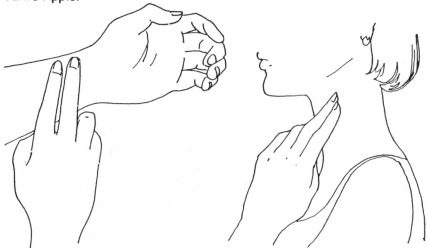

Location of radial pulse   Location of carotid pulse

EVALUATING BODY COMPOSITION

Information about your body proportions, distribution of fatty deposits, and total body fat percentage is needed to help determine your ideal body weight. As will be discussed in Chapter 6, standard height-weight tables can be very misleading since they do not distinguish between weight that is fat and weight that is lean muscle mass. Studies indicate a direct relationship between excess amounts of fat and low levels of physical fitness and a higher risk of cardiovascular disease. A complete analysis of your body composition should therefore include height and body weight, selected girth measurements, and body fat percentage.

Girth Measurement

By measuring the girth of certain areas of the body, you can determine your relative trimness and the relationship of your body proportions to those desired. This is usually an area of high interest since our body proportions determine how we look to others and ourselves.

In order to obtain accurate measurements, you should have another person take your measurements with a standard cloth or plastic tape measure and record them. While being measured, you should stand relaxed and breathe normally with the weight distributed on both feet. The tape measure should be carefully placed around each area so that it remains parallel to the ground and is not applied too tightly. The tissue underneath should not be indented or compressed.

The chart on the next page indicates the sites for your measurements and the recommended girth proportions for men and women. Keep in mind that the recommended proportions can only be used as general guidelines for achieving a trim, well-proportioned body.

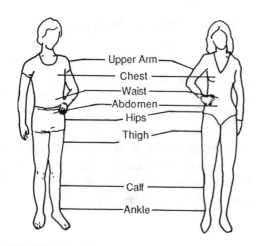

GIRTH
MEASUREMENTS

Site	Recommended Proportion	
	Males	Females
Chest (Bust): at the nipple level	Same as hips	Same as hips
Waist: Below the rib cage above the top of the hip bone (at the minimal abdominal area)	5-7 inches less than chest or hips	10 inches less than bust or hips
Abdomen: Just below the navel, the largest girth between the waist and hips	1 1/2 inches smaller than the chest	2 1/2 inches smaller than bust
Hips: The maximum girth of the buttocks below the hip bone in front	Same as chest	Same as bust
Thigh: An inch or two below the crotch at the largest girth	8-10 inches less than waist	6 inches less than waist
Calf: the largest girth	7-8 inches less than thighs	6-7 inches less than thighs
Ankle: the smallest girth just above the ankle bone	6-7 inches less than calves	5-6 inches less than calves
Upper Arm: the largest girth when the arm is held relaxed with forearm parallel to the floor and palm up	Twice the size of the wrist	Twice the size of the wrist
Wrist: the smallest girth when the arm is held with forearm parallel to the floor and palm up		

Body Fat Measurements

Unfortunately, the most accurate method of measuring body fat is underwater weighing, a complicated process which requires special equipment that may not be available.

A slightly less accurate, but practical, method is the use of skinfold caliper measurements. By measuring the thickness of skinfolds at four specific body sites (the hips, triceps, abdominals, and subscapular), it is relatively easy to obtain an estimate of body fat percentage.

A new technique being used to measure body fat is an electrical impedance unit. These units measure the electrical resistances of the body by detecting changes in electrolyte levels. They work on the principle that lean tissue has a far greater electrolyte content than fat; therefore, the less electrical resistance measured, the more lean tissue a person has and, by inference, the less fat.

According to some authorities, water and bone content vary from person to person and affect body density independently from fat. It is also apparent that exercise (sweating), dehydration, eating, and drinking affect impedance. The readings can be totally off when the body's water compartments are high or low. Dr. Michael Pollock, a noted exercise physiologist, states that he is not certain that electrical impedance will ever match its commercial "hype" because "it overestimates lean individuals and underestimates fat people."

Electrical impedance can also be affected by inherent differences in skin resistance. In addition, day-to-day fluctuations do not pose problems for skinfold testing as they do for electrical impedance testing. The standard error for electrical impedance testing thus far has been much too high. Therefore, at present, only skinfold calipers and underwater weight results are considered reproducible (and therefore scientifically valid).

Lab 6 provides specific information about skinfold measurement as well as norm tables to determine an estimate of your body fat percentage. Percentages are classified in the chart which follows.

BODY FAT CLASSIFICATION

Classification	Percent Fat	
	Male	Female
Very Lean	10%	13%
Lean	11-15%	14-18%
Average	16-19%	19-22%
Fat	20-24%	23-27%
Very Fat	25% over	28% over

Determining Your Target Weight

No doubt one of your primary concerns is how much you should weigh. Chapter 10 points out the problem with using standard weight-height tables that indicate desirable weight based on averages taken from general insurance population statistics. These tables do not consider the percentage of body fat and therefore can be very misleading. A more realistic guide for determining desirable weight is shown in the tables on the next page.

HEIGHT-WEIGHT CHART: MALES

HEIGHT, NO SHOES Feet, Inches	WEIGHT WITHOUT CLOTHES		
	Small Frame	Medium Frame	Large Frame
5 1	107-115	113-124	121-136
5 2	110-118	116-128	124-139
5 3	113-121	119-131	127-143
5 4	116-124	122-134	130-147
5 5	119-128	125-138	133-151
5 6	123-132	129-142	137-156
5 7	127-136	133-147	142-161
5 8	131-140	133-151	146-165
5 9	135-145	141-155	150-169
5 10	139-149	145-160	154-174
5 11	143-153	149-165	159-179
6 0	147-157	153-170	163-184
6 1	151-162	157-175	168-189
6 2	155-166	162-180	173-194
6 3	159-170	167-185	177-199
6 4	163-174	172-190	184-203

HEIGHT-WEIGHT CHART: FEMALES

HEIGHT, NO SHOES Feet, Inches	WEIGHT WITHOUT CLOTHES		
	Small Frame	Medium Frame	Large Frame
4 9	88-90	92-103	100-115
4 10	90-97	94-106	102-118
4 11	92-100	97-109	105-121
5 0	95-103		108-124
5 1	98-106	103-115	111-127
5 2	101-109	106-118	114-130
5 3	104-112	109-122	117-134
5 4	107-115	112-126	121-138
5 5	110-119	116-131	125-142
5 6	114-123	120-135	129-146
5 7	118-127	124-139	133-150
5 8	122-131	128-143	137-154
5 9	126-136	132-147	141-159
5 10	130-140	136-151	145-164
5 11	134-144	140-155	149-169
6 0	138-148	144-159	153-173

The charts above are from Creative Health Products, Plymouth, Michigan.

Once you have determined your percentage of body fat a more accurate calculation of "ideal" or target weight can be made. Use the example which follows to establish your target weight.

EXAMPLE OF TARGET WEIGHT

Fat Weight = $\underset{\text{weight}}{\underline{140}}$ × $\underset{\text{\% fat}}{\underline{.25}}$ = $\underset{\text{lbs. of fat weight}}{\underline{35}}$

Fat Free Weight = $\underset{\text{weight}}{\underline{140}}$ − $\underset{\text{fat weight}}{\underline{35}}$ = $\underset{\text{lbs. of fat free weight}}{\underline{105}}$

Target Weight with Ideal Fat %

Women at 18% fat = $\underset{\text{fat free wt.}}{\underline{105}}$ ÷ 0.82 = $\underset{\text{target weight}}{\underline{128\ \text{lbs.}}}$

men at 12% fat = $\underset{\text{fat free wt.}}{\underline{105}}$ ÷ 0.88 = $\underset{\text{target weight}}{\underline{119\ \text{lbs.}}}$

ESTIMATE OF TARGET WEIGHT

Fat Weight = $\underset{\text{weight}}{\underline{\hspace{2cm}}}$ × $\underset{\text{\% fat}}{\underline{\hspace{2cm}}}$ = $\underset{\text{lbs. of fat weight}}{\underline{\hspace{2cm}}}$

Fat Free Weight = $\underset{\text{weight}}{\underline{\hspace{1.5cm}}}$ − $\underset{\text{fat weight}}{\underline{\hspace{1.5cm}}}$ = $\underset{\text{lbs. of fat free weight}}{\underline{\hspace{1.5cm}}}$

Target Weight with Ideal Fat %

Women at 18% fat = $\underset{\text{fat free wt.}}{\underline{\hspace{2cm}}}$ ÷ 0.82 = $\underset{\text{target weight}}{\underline{\hspace{2cm}}}$

men at 12% fat = $\underset{\text{fat free wt.}}{\underline{\hspace{2cm}}}$ ÷ 0.88 = $\underset{\text{target weight}}{\underline{\hspace{2cm}}}$

EVALUATING FLEXIBILITY

Flexibility is the ability of an individual to move various joints through a maximum range of motion. It is an important aspect of physical fitness, and the lack of flexibility can lead to numerous physical disorders and problems. Basically the loss of flexibility is due to the lack of muscle use. Loss of flexibility can limit one's movements and ability to perform daily tasks as well as recreational activities. No single test can measure flexibility since it is specific to each joint and muscle group. However, the following tests do provide an indication of flexibility for various parts of the body.

Bend and Reach Test

The purpose of this test is to measure the ability to bend your trunk and stretch the muscles of your back and your hamstrings. To perform the test, sit on the floor with your back straight, knees together, and feet flat against a box. As a partner holds your knees straight, reach forward with the arms fully extended, palms down, fingers straight and one hand on top of the other. Hold the position at full extension for at least three seconds. The distance the fingertips reach in relationship to the box is the score — negative scores in front of the box and positive scores beyond the box (and your toes). Ratings for your bend and reach test scores are given below.

Bend and Reach Test

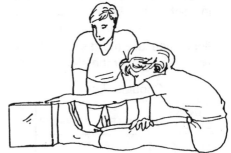

FITNESS CATEGORY	MALES	FEMALES
Superior	> 8	> 8
Excellent	6-7	6-7
Good	4-5	4-5
Average	2-3	2-3
Fair	0-1	0-1
Poor	< 0	< 0

Trunk Extension Test

The purpose of this test is to measure the flexibility of the trunk by arching the back from the prone position. To perform the test, lie prone on the floor, with a partner holding the buttocks and legs down. Interlock your fingers behind your neck with your elbows outward, and raise your chest and head off the floor as high as possible. The distance from the floor to the bottom of your chin is the score. Ratings for the trunk extension test are given below.

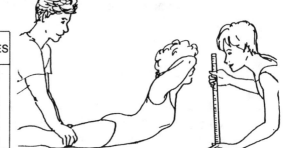

Trunk Extension Test

FITNESS CATEGORY	MALES	FEMALES
Superior	> 24	> 22
Excellent	22-23	20-21
Good	20-21	17-19
Average	18-19	15-16
Fair	16-17	13-14
Poor	< 16	< 13

Shoulder Lift Test

The purpose of this test is to measure the range of motion around the shoulder joint. To perform the test, lie prone on the floor with the chin and forehead touching the floor and the arms extended forward directly in front of the shoulders, with a stick or ruler held in both hands. With a partner holding the buttocks and legs down, and keeping the chin on the floor, measure the distance from the bottom of the stick or ruler to the floor. Ratings for the shoulder lift test follow.

Shoulder Lift

FITNESS CATEGORY	MALES	FEMALES
Superior	> 28	> 27
Excellent	26-27	25-26
Good	24-25	22-24
Average	22-23	19-21
Fair	20-21	17-18
Poor	< 19	< 17

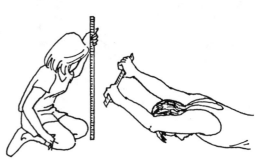

EVALUATING MUSCULAR ENDURANCE

Muscular endurance is a measure of the ability of a specific muscle group to exert force repeatedly or the ability to maintain a given muscle contraction for a period of time. Minimal muscular strength (the ability to apply force) and muscular endurance are needed for everyday tasks, for recreational activities, and to prevent posture problems which are related to muscular weakness, such as lower back pain. Performance on such tests can be affected by one's height, weight, and fatness, but they can provide reasonable estimates of your body strength and muscular endurance.

Bent Knee Sit-Up Test

The purpose of this test is to measure the muscular endurance of the abdominal muscles. To perform this test, lie on your back, face up, with hands on the opposite shoulders. Both feet are placed flat on the floor, with knees flexed at approximately a 90° angle. An assistant holds your feet firmly in place as you sit up to a position with your back perpendicular to the floor and then return to the floor so that your back contacts the floor. The number of sit-ups completed in one minute is the score. Ratings for your sit-up test are below.

FITNESS CATEGORY	BENT KNEE SIT-UP RATINGS MALES (by age)				
	20-29	30-39	40-49	50-59	60-69
Excellent	48 above	40 above	35 above	30 above	25 above
Good	43-47	35-39	30-34	25-29	20-24
Average	37-42	29-34	24-29	19-24	14-19
Fair	33-36	25-28	20-23	15-18	10-13
Poor	0-32	0-24	0-19	0-14	0-9

FITNESS CATEGORY	BENT KNEE SIT-UP RATINGS FEMALES (by age)				
	20-29	30-39	40-49	50-59	60-69
Excellent	44 above	36 above	31 above	26 above	21 above
Good	39-43	31-35	26-30	21-25	16-20
Average	33-38	25-30	19-25	15-20	10-15
Fair	29-32	21-24	16-18	11-14	6-9
Poor	0-28	0-20	0-15	0-10	0-5

Push-up

The purpose of this test is to measure the muscular endurance of the muscles in the arm and shoulder area. To perform this test, assume a front-leaning position on the floor with the hands directly under your shoulders, legs straight and toes tucked to support the body. The body is lowered by bending the elbows until the chin or chest touches the floor and then immediately returned to the starting position. Throughout the test the body is kept in a line from head to toe. The number of correct push-ups one can perform continuously is the score. Ratings for your push-up test follow.

PUSH-UP RATINGS

FITNESS CATEGORY	MALES (by age)					FEMALES	
	20-29	30-39	40-49	50-59	60-69	Rating	Push-Up
Excellent	55 above	45 above	40 above	35 above	30 above	Excellent	27 up
Good	45-54	35-44	30-39	25-34	20-29	Good	19-26
Average	35-44	25-34	20-29	15-24	10-19	Average	12-18
Fair	20-34	15-24	12-19	8-14	5-9	Fair	5-11
Poor	0-19	0-14	0-11	0-7	0-4	Poor	0-4

Static Push-up

The purpose of this test is to serve as an alternate test for the regular push-up test. It is particularly appropriate for those who lack arm strength. To perform the test, assume a front-leaning position on the floor with your hands directly under your shoulders, legs straight and toes tucked to support the body. The body is lowered until the elbows are flexed to a 90° angle or less and held in this position as long as possible. The test is complete when any part of the body touches the floor or the body is not held parallel to the floor. The score is determined by clocking the time in total seconds that the correct position is held. Ratings for your static push-up test follow.

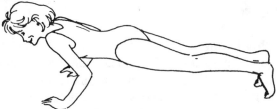

STATIC PUSH-UP RATINGS

MALES		FEMALES	
Rating	Total Time Held	Rating	Total Time Held
Excellent	111 sec. - above	Excellent	35 sec. - above
Good	102-110 sec.	Good	30-34 sec.
Average	97-101 sec.	Average	26-29 sec.
Fair	88-96 sec.	Fair	20-25 sec.
Poor	0-87 sec.	Poor	0-19 sec.

Analyzing the Results

Once you have completed the testing, the results can be used to prepare an individual fitness profile (see Lab 3). This profile will indicate your specific strengths and weaknesses and provide the direction needed to develop an individualized physical improvement program. The next chapter will provide help in designing a program that is safe and effective.

QUESTIONS AND ANSWERS

Is a physical examination necessary before I begin my exercise program?

Although it is advisable to evaluate your physical condition, in most cases people below the age of 35 do not need a physical examination before exercising. If you plan a gradual, sensible exercise program, there are minimal health risks. However, individuals with the following symptoms should seek medical advice: (1) heart trouble, heart murmur; (2) frequent pains or pressure in left or mid-chest area, left neck; (3) often feel faint or have spells of severe dizziness; (4) experience extreme breathlessness after mild exertion; (5) blood pressure too high and not under control; (6) bone or joint problems such as arthritis; (7) over age 35-40 and not accustomed to vigorous exercise; (8) a family history of premature coronary artery disease.

How does smoking affect my fitness level?

Studies definitely show that smokers cannot achieve as high a level of physical fitness as they could if they didn't smoke. Because smoking contributes to a constriction of the blood vessels and a loss in the oxygen-carrying capacity by the blood, the heart rate response will be higher for a given exercise intensity. Individuals who set a goal to achieve optimal fitness but who continue to smoke will automatically fail to reach that goal.

How can I score excellent on one physical fitness test and only fair on another?

Each fitness component — cardiovascular endurance, flexibility, strength, and muscular endurance — is separate and distinct. There is some interrelationship, but achieving a high level in one does not mean you will score high in another. The principle of specificity of training is important to remember; improvement in fitness is specific to the type of training undertaken.

SUGGESTED LABS

Lab 1 - Student Consent Form
Lab 2 - Pre-exercise Medical History Form
Lab 3 - Fitness Profile Chart
Lab 4 - Contract For Change
Lab 5 - Goal Assessment
Lab 6 - Analysis of Body Fat
Lab 7 - Analysis of Body Composition
Lab 12 - Blood Pressure Record

REFERENCES

1. Cooper, Kenneth. *The Aerobics Way.* Bantam Books, New York, 1977.
2. Getchell, Bud. *The Fitness Book.* Benchmark Press, Inc. Indianapolis, Indiana, 1987.
3. Golding, L., Myers, C., and Sinning, W. (eds.) *The Y's Way to Physical Fitness.* National Board of YMCA, Chicago, 1982.
4. Hockey, Robert V. *Physical Fitness — The Pathway to Healthful Living.* C.V. Mosby Co., St. Louis, 1981.
5. Miller, David K. and Allen, T. Earl. *Fitness : A Lifetime Commitment.* Burgess Publishing Co., Minneapolis, 1986.
6. Stokes, R., Moore, A., and Moore C. *Fitness: The New Wave.* Hunter Textbooks, Inc., Winston-Salem, NC, 1988.

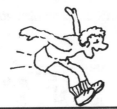

Chapter Three

Getting Started
TRAINING PROGRAMS

Now that you have gained an understanding of your current fitness level, you are ready to develop a program that will help you reach your highest level of fitness. Your optimal level relates to your particular interests, needs, and abilities. Each of us is different, but regardless of our previous experience, disease or disability, all of us can improve our health and strive for optimal fitness. It is not important to compare yourself to others — seek to achieve the highest level possible for you.

Success in reaching this level will depend to a large extent on the program you utilize. Unfortunately many people with good intentions become frustrated and fall short of their goal because of basic fallacies in their training program. By observing certain principles and guidelines you can safely engage in a program that will provide maximum results.

PRINCIPLES OF TRAINING

Three basic principles will determine the effectiveness of any training program. Understanding and applying these principles is essential to developing a program which will produce improvement. In addition, following these principles will enable you to safely engage in a progressive training program. These three principles are **overload, progression and specificity.**

Overload

Overload occurs when increased demands are made upon the body. These demands cause the body to adapt which results in an improvement in physical condition. Overload can be accomplished in three general ways:

1. **Frequency.** By increasing how often one exercises, the number of times per day and/or week that an activity is performed. Exercise must be performed on a regular basis if it is to be effective. Hopefully exercise will become a part of your daily lifestyle; however, benefits can be achieved with at least **three workouts per week**. The workouts should be spaced throughout the week rather than on consecutive days. A frequency of four or five times per week will produce a greater caloric expenditure.

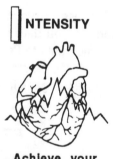

F REQUENCY

OCTOBER

						1
2	3	4	5	6	7	8
9	10	11	12	13	14	15
16	17	18	19	20	21	22
23	24	25	26	27	28	29
30	31					

**At least
3 times per week**

2. **Intensity.** By increasing the difficulty of an exercise, such as increasing the speed of a run, amount of weight lifted, or distance stretched. Exercise must be strenuous enough to require more effort than usual. As the body adapts to this workload, an increased demand can be placed upon it. The intensity needed to produce improvement will vary depending upon the current physical condition of the individual. In a poorly conditioned person, walking may be strenuous enough to produce a training effect.

I NTENSITY

**Achieve your
target heart rate**

3. **Time (or duration).** By increasing the length of each training session. In order to be effective, exercise must be maintained for a significant length of time. A 30-minute workout allows for sufficient warm-up and cool-down with at least 15 minutes at the target heart rate level. If you only exercise

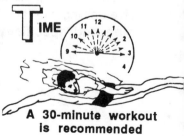

T IME

**A 30-minute workout
is recommended**

three times a week, the total duration should be extended by 10-15 minutes to increase the caloric expenditure for the week. Exercise duration and intensity are directly related. Therefore, an activity performed at a higher intensity can be done for a shorter duration (with 15 minutes a day at a higher intensity as the minimum duration). The duration must be increased for those activities, such as walking, done at a lower intensity.

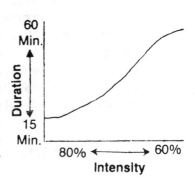

Progression

Progression is a combination of adaptation and overload. Adaptation refers to the body's ability to adapt to stress. This means that as you force your body to work harder, it will eventually adjust in order to work more efficiently. Since the body adjusts to stress, the amount of work must be periodically increased in order for improvement to occur. For example, if you began an exercise program that involved running one mile a day in eight minutes, you would probably find the workout stressful. You would, therefore, improve your cardiovascular function for the next several weeks if you continued the eight-minute rate. But if you continued to perform at that level (i.e., run the same distance in the same time), cardiovascular improvement would stop and adaptation would occur. To continue improving, you would have to increase the stress on your cardiovascular system; and, therefore, the overload principle would go into effect again. In a few weeks or months, additional overload would again have to be added.

Specificity

The specificity principle implies that the improvements made in training are specific to the type of training undertaken. For example, a strength program will develop strength, but not an appreciable amount of endurance. Another illustration is the person who has trained adequately for a sport such as swimming, but when that person participates in basketball or some other sport, he or she quickly becomes fatigued during play and muscle-sore later. Each activity requires specific demand, and doing the event is the best way to train for the event.

Finally, it must be realized that no two people are alike. Everyone does not progress or improve at the same rate. Each person will respond to the training program at his or her own unique rate. Concentrate on other changes you are achieving and do not compare your progress with that of others. If you are observing the principles and guidelines noted in this chapter, you will eventually achieve your optimal level of fitness. Keep working but be patient!

DETERMINING TARGET HEART RATE

In order to reach the necessary intensity, it has been noted that you exercise in your target heart rate zone. For most young adults, a target heart rate between 150-170 beats per minute will achieve this intensity. Older adults may only need to achieve a rate between 130-140 beats per minute to reach their target heart rate zone. To determine your specific target heart rate you should follow these easy steps.

220	(MHR The maximum heart rate you can achieve during exercise)
- _____	(Your age — the MHR decreases as one gets older)
= _____	(Your MHR)
- _____	(Your resting heart rate)
= _____	(Heart rate reserve)
X ___.75___	(75% workout intensity — between 60 and 80% is recommended)
= _____	
+ _____	(Your resting heart rate)
= _____	Target Heart Rate at the 75% level

By determining your target heart rate zone, you can be certain you are achieving an intensity high enough to benefit from the workout and yet not be pushing yourself too hard. Exercising within your target zone should not make you feel greatly uncomfortable. If you feel overly tired, try working at a lower rate until you are ready to progress to a higher zone.

Since it is difficult to count your pulse while performing a vigorous exercise, try counting it immediately after the workout. By counting the beats for 10 seconds and multiplying by 6, you will have a relatively accurate estimate of your heart rate during exercise. With practice you will know how you feel when you reach your target heart rate and frequent checks will not be necessary.

THE EXERCISE SESSION

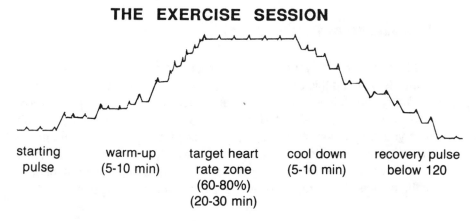

| starting pulse | warm-up (5-10 min) | target heart rate zone (60-80%) (20-30 min) | cool down (5-10 min) | recovery pulse below 120 |

The above diagram illustrates the typical pattern one should follow during each individual exercise session. It is important to develop the habit of including all steps — the elimination of any step, such as the cool-down, could lead to problems.

THE WARM-UP

The purpose of the warm-up phase is to prepare the body for the increased stress which will be placed upon it. If possible, the warm-up activity should relate specifically to the exercise to be performed. The next chapter provides specific guidelines for the warm-up.

THE WORKOUT

It is important to observe the principle of overload and strive to reach the target heart rate, during an aerobic exercise session.

MONITORING AND EVALUATING THE WORKOUT

As you participate in an aerobic exercise program, there are certain guidelines to be followed when monitoring your body's response to exercise and in evaluating the effectiveness of the program. We all want to know that our time and effort are being well spent.

Pre-exercise Pulse Check

It is wise to check your resting pulse before starting the exercise session. By charting this on a regular basis you can see if your heart rate is declining, which is an indication of an effective aerobics program. If you happen to notice an elevated resting heart rate one day, it could mean that you are under stress due to a lack of sleep, anxiety, emotional problems or over-training. This may also be a sign that the workout needs to be shortened or the intensity lowered. In this case, careful monitoring of the exercise heart rate and recovery heart rate are suggested.

Exercise Heart Rate

Monitoring the heart rate during the exercise session is essential in order to measure the intensity of the workout. Remember, the workout should cause the heart rate to increase to the target heart rate zone and stay there for at least 15 minutes. The heart rate should also be checked after starting the workout and at ten-minute intervals. In this way you can be relatively sure when your target heart rate is reached, whether the heart rate is being maintained at the appropriate level, and how long your level is maintained. When taking the exercise heart rate, you should continue to move around (easy jog, walk, cycle slowly, etc.) in order to prevent the blood from pooling in the extremities as the pulse is counted.

Talk Test

A practical way to monitor the intensity of your workout is the talk test. As you do aerobic exercise the heart and respiratory rates increase to meet the body's demands for increased oxygen. However, aerobic exercise should be done at an intensity that will allow a steady supply of oxygen to be delivered for that activity to be sustained and at the same time enable you to talk without difficulty. If you cannot get enough air to carry on a conversation, the exercise is probably too strenuous and should be decreased. The talk test is a good guide to determine whether the intensity is too high, but if you are in doubt as to whether it is high enough, a pulse check should be taken.

Perceived Exertion

As you get into an exercise program, it is important to recognize your body's response to the activity. By asking yourself the following questions you will be able to judge the intensity of your workout: How rapid is my rate of breathing? How much am I perspiring? Am I able to talk? How tired do I feel? Are my muscles fatiguing?

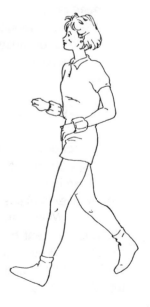

By checking your pulse at various times and comparing it to your perceived exertion, you will soon be able to judge the intensity of your workout without stopping to take your pulse. An occasional spot check will be sufficient to verify that you are achieving the target heart rate zone.

Using Hand Weights

One way to increase the workout for your heart and lungs while walking, running, jogging, or aerobic dancing is to carry hand weights. By using light weights in each hand and swinging your arms while doing the exercise, you can increase the work you are doing. The type of arm exercise you do, can vary depending upon your specific goal, but the best guide to the

effect of using the weights is your heart rate. If you do not notice a difference in your heart rate, you may want to consider using heavier weights
or making the arm movements more vigorous.

The advantage of carrying a weight as you workout is that it increases
the amount of energy used, and therefore you do not need to walk significantly faster or jog to increase your heart rate. The following guidelines should be observed when using hand weights:

1. Be certain you warm up the arm muscles before the session.
2. Start gradually — the key is to use light weights (no more than half a
    pound and increase by half pound increments) and to carry the same
    weight on each side. You may be surprised at how little weight is
    needed for the increase you desire.
3. Grip the weights securely but not too tightly.
4. Use controlled movements rather than wild swinging action. Make
    certain you are using the muscles to maintain control and if you are
    pumping your arms, push your fist no higher than shoulder height
    with every swing.
5. Remember to check your pulse rate — you may be able to lower your
    pace and intensity due to the effect of the weights in increasing your
    heart rate.
6. The use of weights during a high-impact aerobic class is not recom-
    mended because the movements are generally too fast for control.
7. If you have chronic back pain, it may be best to avoid using weights.

THE COOL-DOWN

The cool-down allows the body to gradually return to its starting point.
For this, a simple slowing down of the exercise can be used. The gradual
cool down is extremely important to prevent possible pooling of blood in
the lower extremities—a common occurrence after vigorous endurance
exercise. Without the contraction of the muscles in the extremities, the
blood is not sent back to the heart and brain, and may cause one to
experience dizziness or faintness. In addition, light stretching assists in
cooling the body and helps prevent soreness from unaccustomed use of
muscles. This is also an excellent time to improve flexibility.

The Recovery Heart Rate

One final check on the quality of any exercise session can be made by checking the recovery heart rate. If the intensity and duration of your workout were appropriate, your heart rate five minutes after the exercise should be below 120 beats per minute. A heart rate higher than this indicates that perhaps the intensity of the program should be lowered and/or that the duration should be less. Remember, your goal is to have an effective program but one that is not greatly uncomfortable — one that you can enjoy!

Now that you are aware of the principles for an aerobic session, you are ready to establish your specific program. The following guidelines may assist you in planning the most appropriate one for you.

SETTING UP AN EXERCISE PROGRAM

Factors to consider in selecting an activity:
- age
- health status
- present level of fitness
- previous activity and training experience
- psychological factors and motivation
- goals

Keep the following in mind as you set up your exercise program:
- Set realistic goals
- Keep a record of workouts (time, distance, heart rate, etc.).
- Plan for obstacles (weather, time, soreness, etc.).
- Use appropriate training techniques to maximize the effect.
- A lower level of intensity is suggested for those with a lower initial level of fitness.
- The less fit, middle-aged, and older participants should take more time to warm up.
- The initial level of exercise should be maintained for a longer period of time for the unfit participant (2-4 weeks). After this time, a steady progression can be utilized.

QUESTIONS AND ANSWERS

Does missing a few sessions cause me to lose my fitness?

One does not lose all the gains of an exercise program by missing a few days. However, when you begin exercising again you should start at a lower level. Depending on the number of days you missed and how you feel while exercising, it is suggested you begin at half to two-thirds your usual exercise level. Once you have missed the days, don't worry about them — just get back on schedule and work toward achieving your goal.

Should I join a health spa?

Before making what could be an expensive membership commitment to a health spa or sport club, you should consider the following factors:
1. Numerous abuses have been reported. Deceptive advertising, high pressure sales tactics, misrepresentation in sales presentations, and restrictive and unfair contract cancellation policies are a few.
2. Membership is a long-term commitment and to get your money's worth you have to work out regularly at least two to three times a week.
3. If the site is located more than 20 minutes from your home, don't join.
4. Drop in during the hours you would probably be attending to see if over-crowding will be a problem.
5. Check to be sure the equipment is adequate and the type you need, i.e., weights, exercise bicycles, treadmill.
6. Ask about the instructors and check their credentials and qualifications.
7. Examine the written contract carefully before signing it.
8. Make certain similar facilities are not already available at a lower cost or free at a nearby school, college, YWCA or YMCA.

How will I know if I have exceeded the safe limits for exercise?

There are several warning signs which indicate you are over-exercising and should reduce the intensity of the workout: excessive heart rate, labored breathing, pale skin, flushness, and a prolonged heart rate recovery time after exercising.

Any of the following signs indicate that exercise should be stopped immediately because the participant may be in danger: difficulty in breathing (not just deep breathing); loss of coordination; dizziness; tightness in the chest. If the participant exhibits any of these danger signs, he/she should seek medical advice before continuing with the exercise program.

What differences in the results of training will there be between men and women?

The following physiological differences will affect the training potential of women: (1) smaller heart; (2) slightly lower hemoglobin level; (3) less total muscle mass than men. The effect of the first two differences is a lower potential maximum oxygen uptake because less oxygen will be available to the cells during exercise. The effect of the third difference is less total body strength for women compared to men. In spite of these differences, men and women can participate in the same types of training programs and both can realize improvement in their level of physical fitness.

What causes the "stitch in the side"?

A "stitch" or sudden, sharp pain in the side or upper part of the abdomen, is a form of muscle cramp. Physicians now believe that a cramp occurs in the diaphragm muscle due to the blood supply being cut off by the pressure from the lungs above and the abdomen below during exercise. The muscle goes into a spasm when it is unable to get enough oxygen. You can help prevent a "stitch" by strengthening your diaphragm and abdominal muscles. To relieve the pain, slow down and push your fingers deep into the site of the pain, just below the last rib on the upper right part of the abdomen. Now bend forward and exhale, puckering your lips. When the pain disappears you can continue exercising.

What special precautions should I take on a hot humid day?

The body needs time to adapt to hot weather conditions. Even though you might be physically fit, you can only increase your tolerance to heat by exercising regularly in hot weather. Therefore, the following steps are recommended:

1. Plan your workouts for the coolest part of the day, such as early morning or early evening after the sun has gone down.
2. Cut back on your workouts — duration and intensity — until you become adapted to the heat.
3. Drink plenty of fluids — especially water.
4. Dress in light-weight, loose-fitting clothing.
5. Never wear rubberized clothing, plastic suits, sweatshirts or sweat pants.

What are the symptoms of heat exhaustion and heat stroke?

The usual symptoms of heat exhaustion include abnormally low body temperature, dizziness, headache, nausea and sometimes, mental confusion. Symptoms of heat stroke include dizziness, headache, thirst, nausea, muscle cramps, and three important symptoms: sweating stops, a dangerously high body temperature develops, and unconsciousness frequently occurs. This condition can be very serious. Since excessive body temperature can cause brain damage and even death, medical attention is critical for heat stroke.

What are the dangers of rubberized or plastic clothing?

Many people in their eagerness to lose weight mistake water loss caused by excessive sweating with fat loss. The excessive dehydration caused by wearing rubberized or plastic clothing can be extremely Dangerous and does not contribute to a permanent weight loss. The wearing of such clothing causes the body temperature to rise to a potentially dangerous level because the sweat cannot evaporate and evaporation is the body's cooling mechanism. As the temperature continues to rise, sweating increases, leading to excessive water loss.

What causes muscle soreness?

Most muscle soreness occurs between 24-48 hours after the exercise. Although the specific cause is not known, it appears to be due to small tears in the muscle or the connective tissue around the muscle. Previous theories linked the soreness to a buildup of lactic acid in the muscle during sustained activity. In any case, you can help prevent the pain and stiffness by proper warm-up and cool-down, by gradually getting into your exercise program, by progressing slowly, and by avoiding ballistic or bouncing-type stretching exercises.

How should I dress on extremely cold days?

It is important to dress appropriately when exercising outside on cold days. Generally the following rules should be observed:
1. Wear one layer less of clothing than you would if you were outside but not exercising.
2. Wear several layers of light clothing rather than one heavy layer.
3. Protect your hands by wearing old mittens, gloves, or cotton socks.
4. Wear a head covering. Up to 40% of your body's heat is lost through the neck and head.

It is also suggested that a brief warm-up before going outside is beneficial.

Does it really matter which exercises I choose to do?

All exercises are not the same. Not only do some exercises burn more calories per minute, but exercises provide benefits which are specific to the type of exercise. For instance, stretching exercises will only contribute to an increase in flexibility — not to strength or endurance. The exercises requiring continuous activity and involving large muscle groups will provide the greatest caloric expenditure. Therefore, you must select exercises which meet your needs — whether it is for a specific fitness component or for weight control.

Should I drink one of the special exercise drinks—Gatorade, ERG, Quick Kick, etc.?

You should first understand that sweat is 99.1% water and therefore the body is not losing a significant quantity of the electrolytes (sodium, potassium, magnesium, calcium, and phosphate) which are contained in these drinks. During heavy sweating you actually lose so much water that the remaining electrolytes are more concentrated. It is also important to understand that the replacement of lost fluid is slowed significantly when the ingested fluid contains sugar (whether in the form of glucose, fructose, or sucrose). Therefore, if you do drink commercial preparations, they should be diluted to speed their absorption.

Is a protein meal the best source of energy before a workout or athletic event?

No. Actually, protein digestion is more complex and takes longer than carbohydrate digestion. Therefore, the best meal would be one with a high level of complex carbohydrates. These are broken down slowly and provide the body with energy for a longer period of time. In addition, carbohydrates are stored in the liver and muscles in the form of glycogen which is then readily available for conversion into glucose when extra energy is needed.

SUGGESTED LABS

Lab 10 Target Heart Rate Zone
Lab 11 Exercise Recording Form

REFERENCES

1. Garrison, L., Leslie, P., and Blackmore, D. *Fitness and Figure Control.* Mayfield Publishing Co., Palo Alto, California, 1981.
2. Getchell, Bud. *The Fitness Book.* Benchmark Press Inc., Indianapolis, Indiana, 1987.
3. Golding, L., Myers, C., and Sinning, W. (eds.). *The Y's Way to Physical Fitness.* National Board of YMCA, Chicago, 1982.
4. Sharkey, Brian. *Physiology of Fitness.* Human Kinetics Pub., Champaign, Illinois, 1979.
5. Stokes, R., Moore, A., and Moore, C. *Fitness: The New Wave.* Hunter Textbooks Inc., Winston-Salem, NC, 1988.
6. U.S. Dept. of Health and Human Services. *Exercise and Your Heart.* U. S. Government Printing Office, Washington, DC, 1981.

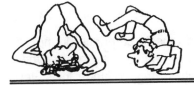

Chapter Four

Stretch Out and Shape Up
DEVELOPING FLEXIBILITY

Flexibility is an important component of fitness that increases the extensibility of muscles, tendons, and ligaments. Each person, depending upon personal needs, must have a reasonable amount of flexibility to perform everyday activities. The range of motion at any joint may vary, depending on the shape of the bones and cartilage in the joint and the length of the muscles and ligaments that cross it. Exactly how much flexibility any one person should have is not known; however, there are test standards that give some guidelines as to the amount of flexibility most desirable for various age groups and sex. Too much flexibility in certain joints may make a person more susceptible to injury and make the joint susceptible to dislocation (5).

Flexibility is important in helping prevent injuries in areas of the body such as the calf and the lower back. Thousands of people suffer from lower back problems which can be resolved with a well-balanced flexibility program (3). A good flexibility program includes stretches for the calf, the lower back, the hip flexors and the quadriceps. Because these muscles are most frequently used during aerobic exercise, they should be thoroughly stretched before and after an aerobic workout. When stretching for the purpose of increasing flexibility, you should try to lengthen the muscle to increase its elasticity.

Increased elasticity and flexibility enhance physical and athletic skills. Flexibility facilitates performance skills and assists in coordinated and aesthetically pleasing movement. For example, dancers spend many hours stretching abductor and adductor muscles for performing leaps and turns; swimmers work to develop shoulder and ankle flexibility for powerful strokes; and runners develop flexibility to improve and lengthen their stride. Without flexibility, highly skilled performance is almost impossible.

Stretching exercises appear to relieve muscle soreness during and after a workout. There are two types of pain related to exercise. One is the pain immediately after exercising, which may continue for several hours after exercise ceases. The other is a pain that occurs 24 to 48 hours after the exercise session is completed. One theory suggests that static stretching (stretching without bouncing) helps relieve the pain of tight, contracted, over-extended muscles. Stretching exercises are also recommended to women suffering from dysmenorrhea (painful menstruation) (5). By stretching the muscles in the pelvic and hip area, the discomfort in the lower back can be minimized.

In addition to relieving muscle soreness, stretching also appears to decrease the intensity and incidence of musculotendinous and joint injury (3). Although this theory has not been proven, it does appear that increased flexibility will help prevent or minimize injuries when the muscles and joints are accidentally overstretched. Therefore, strong, flexible, well-stretched muscles can help prevent injuries during aerobic exercise.

To increase flexibility, one must overload the muscles by stretching them beyond their normal range of movement. Research suggests stretching about ten percent beyond the normal range. When designing your flexibility program, there are special factors to consider. Flexibility may vary with each of the following:

1. Age — From about age twenty, flexibility declines unless you engage in a regular program of flexibility exercises.
2. Sex — Because of their greater muscle bulk, men often have more difficulty developing and maintaining flexibility.
3. Stress factors — illness, lack of sleep, final exams, and other stressful situations may contribute to tight muscles.
4. Time of the day — Muscles tend to be tighter in the morning than in the afternoon and evening.
5. Arthritic joint disease — Disease may prohibit some movements.
6. Injury —May cause some inflexibility in muscles and joints.
7. Obesity — Being overweight makes it difficult to stretch properly.
8. Fitness level —Those who are physically active tend to be more flexible than their sedentary counterparts.

TYPES OF STRETCHING

There are three basic types of stretching techniques: static stretch, ballistic stretch and proprioceptive neuromuscular facilitator (PNF).

Static stretching is performed slowly with controlled movement which minimizes the amount of pain experienced and thus lowers the risk of tearing muscle tissue. An effective method of static stretching is to hold the muscle in the maximal stretch position from 10 to 60 seconds. As flexibility improves, the amount of time held may be increased. The muscle that is being stretched should be aligned to reinforce the lengthening effect of the exercise. If severe pain is experienced, change the position of your body or discontinue the stretch.

Ballistic stretching, as compared to static stretch, uses momentum to achieve flexibility. The inherent danger in this technique is that the uncontrolled, sudden movement may stretch the muscle farther than it is capable of being stretched. Most aerobic exercise instructors avoid this type of stretching.

The third technique is the proprioceptive neuromuscular facilitator method. This stretch method relies on reflex mechanisms to increase the range of motion. It requires the assistance of another person to apply controlled force to increase the angle of stretch. This method is used primarily in the rehabilitation of injuries.

STRETCHING TECHNIQUES

Static Waist Stretch
Begin standing with proper alignment. Slowly stretch the upper body diagonally up and to the side. The knees should be flexed and the shoulders relaxed. Repeat the stretch on both sides of the body.

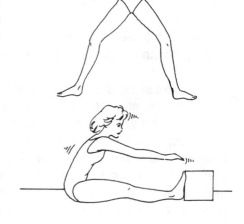

Ballistic Stretch
Legs extended, feet flexed. Stretch forward using a bouncing, percussive motion.

Proprioceptive Neuromuscular Facilitation
Sitting, the partner assists in stretching an isolated muscle or muscle group. A contraction-relaxation approach is used for this stretching.

To get the optimal benefits from a static stretch program, follow these guidelines:
1. Use proper alignment when stretching muscles.
2. Hold the stretch for 10-60 seconds depending on your flexibility fitness level.
3. Stretch to the point of slight discomfort.
4. Be sensitive to the limitations of your body.
5. Strengthen the muscles you stretch.
6. Avoid locking or hyperextending the joints of the body.
7. Stretch every day for maximum benefits and results.

WARM-UP

To achieve the optimal level of flexibility, you should warm the muscles of the body before stretching. Warm-up exercises should be followed by flexibility exercises. With proper warm-up, the body temperature should increase and cause muscle extensibility. The benefits of warm-up activities include the following:
1. Increased blood flow to the muscles resulting in more oxygen and nutrients being readily available.
2. Higher rate of oxygen exchange between blood and muscles.
3. Reduced chances of muscle, tendon and ligament injury.
4. More efficient muscle contraction due to faster nerve impulse transmission.
5. Decreased muscle tension.
6. Improved reaction time.
7. Less post-exercise muscle soreness.
8. A psychological readiness for exercise.

An effective warm-up should include the following:
1. Light calisthenic activities with some dynamic flexibility exercises.
2. Movements similar to those that will be performed during actual workout.
3. Exercises that gradually and smoothly lead into more intense and vigorous activity.

The amount of time that is spent on warm-up depends on the fitness level of the class, the room temperature, and the type of class. A thorough warm-up can provide favorable results and help to protect you from injuries. The intensity and duration of the warm-up must be individualized to fit the needs of the students and the type of activity.

Warm-up Stretches

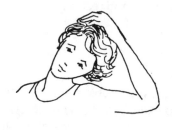

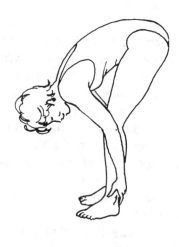

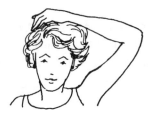

Neck Stretch
Gently place the hand on the head and pull to the side. Keep the shoulders down and relaxed.

Forward Stretch
Stand with feet shoulder width apart. Knees flexed. Gently roll the body down until you feel a slight tension in the back of the legs. Hold the stretch and repeat the sequence.

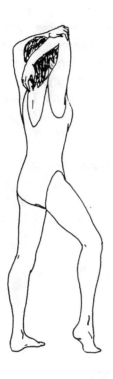

Upper Body Stretch

Place both arms behind the head and gently apply resistance with opposite hand to elbow. Stretch until you feel a slight tension. Release and repeat several times.

Low Lunge Stretch

Lunge forward with the knee over the toes, hips square. Gently press the hip toward the floor until you experience a stretch in the front of the hip and thigh. Relax and repeat on the other side.

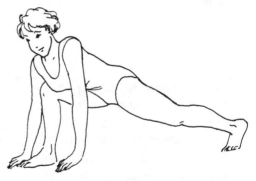

COOL-DOWN

The cool-down can be thought of as a warm-up in reverse. While warm-up activities increase the heart rate, cool-down exercise helps the body make the transition from intense activity to rest. Cooling down also makes the body feel good and helps prevent muscle soreness. Cool-down exercises can be similar to those used in warming up. Low-intensity, stretching activities help to bring the heart rate to a pre-existing level and allow the blood flow to return to the heart safely and efficiently.

The cool-down is an ideal time for concentrating on flexibility. The body is warm and the muscles are most receptive to safe stretching. During cool-down, the heart rate should drop below 120 beats and profuse sweating should cease. When the cool-down is completed, there should be a feeling of invigoration and relaxation.

Cool-down Stretches

Hip Abductor Stretch
Sit with a straight spine, shoulders relaxed. Place one leg over the extended opposite leg. Press gently against the leg. Hold the stretch. Repeat on the other side.

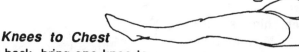

Knees to Chest
Lie on back, bring one knee to the chest, extend the other leg. Gently press the leg into the chest. Alternate legs and then bring both legs in together. Hold, then relax the stretch and repeat several times.

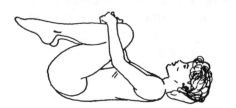

Gluteal Stretch

Sit straight, one leg extended in front of the body. Gently bring the other leg into the body until a stretch is felt in the back of the upper leg and/or outside the hip. Repeat the stretch on the other side.

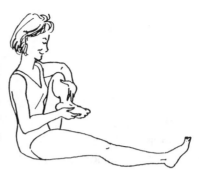

Thigh Stretch

Lie on your side, torso aligned. Grasp the ankle of the leg on top and pull gently until you feel a stretch in the front of the thigh. Do not arch the back and keep the knee pointed forward. Release and repeat on the other side.

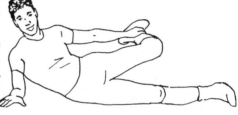

Hamstring Stretch

Lie on your back with one knee bent and gently bring the other leg toward the chest as you straighten the leg. Relax and repeat on the other leg.

Chest Stretch

Place one leg in front of the other in a lunge position. Clasp hands behind the back, extend the arms up and out, squeezing the shoulder blades together. Hold the stretch. Relax and repeat the stretch.

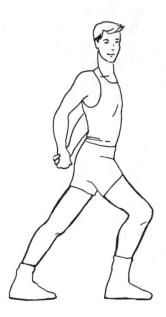

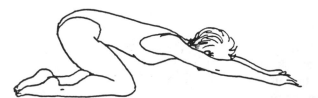

Total Back Stretch

Kneel on the floor, extend both arms in front of the body. Align the spine, press the chest to the floor and hold the position.

QUESTIONS AND ANSWERS

When I stretch, I feel very tight in one leg, but flexible and loose in the other. Why?

Flexibility varies in each joint and on each side of the body. Recognize this and stretch accordingly.

Is it true that men are less flexible than women?

Generally speaking, yes. Men tend to be tighter because of muscle bulk and muscle and joint structure.

What is better, ballistic or static stretching?

Although there is some controversy about this issue, static stretching is preferable because it is safer.

If I do aerobic and strength training programs, do I still need to stretch?

Most definitely. Aerobic activity generally tightens many of the major muscle groups and the lower back, so stretching is an important part of a balanced exercise program.

Should I always stretch to the point of pain?

Stretch until you feel a tension in the muscle indicating that you are extending past the point of comfort. Be sensitive to the kind of pain that you feel; when it becomes intense you should stop stretching and begin again.

How do I stretch correctly?

Correct stretching requires that you hold the stretch position until the tension in the muscle releases. This can take about twenty seconds to one minute.You should stretch your muscles just slightly beyond the point of fatigue.

Should I warm up before I stretch?

Yes. You should raise your body temperature and get your muscles in a ready-to-exercise state. This can be done with light calisthenics, or stepping in place or walking for 3 to 5 minutes.

When is the best time to stretch?

The best time to stretch your muscles is after exercise when the muscles are warm.

Why is it important to cool down?

The cool-down is important because it provides a safe return from high intensity exercise to rest.

REFERENCES

1. Alter, J. *Stretch and Strengthen*. Houghton Mifflin Co., Boston, 1986.
2. Alter, J. *Surviving Exercise*. Houghton Mifflin Co., Boston, 1983.
3. Alter, M. *The Science of Stretching*. Human Kinetics, Champaign, IL, 1988.
4. Brehm, B.A. "Cool Down Physiology," *Fitness Management* 11 (9) 15,1988.
5. Corbin, C. and Lindsey, R. *Concepts of Physical Fitness with Laboratories*. Wm.C. Brown Co.,Philadelphia,1988.
6. Elam, R. "Best Warmup and Cool Down Stretches," *Shape* 7 (4) 55,1988.
7. Etyre, B.R. and Lee, E.J. "Chronic and Acute Flexibility of Men and Women Using Three Different Stretching Techniques," *Research Quarterly for Exercise and Sport* 59 (9) (3) 222,1988.
8. Hoeger, W.K.*Principles and Labs for Physical Fitness and Wellness*. Morton Publishing Co., Englewood, CO, 1988.
9. Miller, D.K. and Allen, T.E. *Fitness, A Lifetime Commitment*. Burgess Publishing Co., Minneapolis, 1986.
10. Shellock, F.J. "Physiological Benefits of Warmup," *The Physician and Sportsmedicine* 11 (10) 117, 1983.
11. Stamford, B. "Flexibility and Stretching," *The Physician and Sportsmedicine* 2 (9) 171, 1984.
12. Stokes, R., Moore, A. and Moore, C. *Fitness: The New Wave*. Hunter Textbooks Inc. Winston-Salem, NC, 1988.
13. Trapp, D.E. and Hollifield N.L. *Aerobic Dance: A Focus On Fitness*. Burgess Press, Minneapolis, MN, 1986.

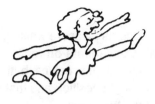

Chapter Five

Find Your Beat
AEROBIC FITNESS

The term *aerobic* means "in the presence of oxygen" and suggests that an exercise program increases the supply and use of oxygen. This ability to supply and utilize oxygen is important because oxygen is essential for the body to sustain life and function efficiently.

To increase work capacity, the circulatory and respiratory systems must be trained to deliver oxygen more readily. This can be done by overloading the system and requiring the system to respond to greater than normal demands. The systematic overloading of the circulatory system represents a primary standard for determining whether or not an exercise program is aerobic. The criteria which must be met by an exercise program to be aerobic are as follows:

1. It must involve large muscle groups in rhythmic, dynamic contraction.
2. It must be performed at an intensity which overloads the circulatory system beyond normal demands.
3. It must require that the body deliver large amounts of oxygen to the cells for a prolonged period of time.
4. It must be performed four or more times per week for a moderately active person to achieve an improved fitness level. Three exercise periods per week will improve cardiorespiratory fitness for the sedentary individual, and will maintain a current level of fitness for the moderately active person.

Following are brief descriptions of basic exercise programs for achieving aerobic fitness. You may want to experiment with more than one program and utilize a variety to achieve your goal. Select the program which is enjoyable to you. Find your beat!

WALKING

Technique

Remember, walking for fitness is not the same as pleasure walking. No shuffling, strolling or sauntering is allowed! Concentrate on really using your muscles (and contracting them) — the feet, thighs, calves, buttocks, diaphragm, etc. Make certain you are in an upright position and that your entire foot is placed on the ground — heel first, then toes.

Procedure

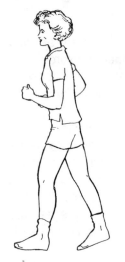

1. Start slowly and use the first 3-5 minutes as a warm-up. Increase your pace gradually.
2. Try to get in rhythm with a natural, effortless motion.
3. Use a stride that is natural for you but lengthen your stride gradually to increase the speed of your walking.
4. As you quicken your pace, thrust harder with your legs, increase your arm swing, and breathe naturally.

Suggested Program

FITNESS CATEGORY = AVERAGE

Starter Walking Program (2)

Week	Frequency/Wk	Distance	Time
	Days	Miles	min:sec
1	3	2.0	34:16
2	3	2.0	34:16
3	3	2.0	30:00
4	4	2.0	30:00
5	3	2.5	37:50
6	3	2.5	37:50

JOGGING

Technique

Select comfortable, loose-fitting clothing (no rubberized suits). Proper shoes are essential — those with well protected heel or arch support, firm soles, pliable tops, and proper fit. Run "tall" and keep your head up. Hold arms slightly away from the body and bend at the elbows. Either land first on the heel of the foot and rock forward to the ball of the foot or land on the entire bottom of the foot. Keep your steps short by letting the foot strike the grounds beneath the knee. Breathe deeply through your mouth and nose while jogging.

Procedure

1. Begin slowly—perhaps a walking program is needed first.
2. When starting, make certain you are com-fortable and can talk with the person next to you.
3. Pace yourself and stay at the same level for a longer period if it continues to challenge you.

Suggested Program: start by walking, then walk and run or run as necessary.

Under 30 years of age (2)

Week	Frequency (Per Week)	Distance (miles)	Time (min.)
1	3	2.0	32:00
2	3	2.0	30:30
3	3	2.0	27:00
4	3	2.0	26:00
5	3	1.0	25:00
6	3	2.0	24:30
7	3	2.0	24:00
8	3	2.0	22:00
9	3	2.0	21:00
10	3	2.0	19:00
11	4	2.0	18:00
12	3	2.0	< 18:00
		or 2.5	< 22:00

ROPE SKIPPING

Technique

Select a suitable rope: a #10 sash cord, commercial jump rope, or any piece of rope long enough to reach the armpits when held beneath the feet. Use small circular movements of your arms; use mainly the hands and wrists. Keep jumps small, spring mostly from ankles, land as lightly as possible and allow just enough room for the rope to pass under your feet.

Procedure

1. Start with easy jumping from foot to foot as if running in place.
2. Next, try jumping twice for every turn of the rope — once over the rope and then a small bounce while the rope passes overhead.
3. Try to keep your jumps continuous and jump only once for each turn of the rope.
4. Advance to hopping, running, kicking, rope crosses, and moving forward and backward.
5. If you tire too quickly, walk or jog slowly in place and then continue jumping.

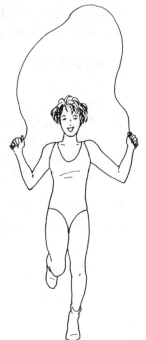

Suggested Program

Week

1 - Jump 5 two-minute series (stretch between each series).

2 - Jump 5 three-minute series (stretch between each series).

3 - Jump 3 five-minute series with stretching.

4 - Jump 2 seven-minute series with stretching.

5 - Jump 10 minutes, stretch, then jump 5 minutes.

6 - Jump 15 minutes and stretch.

CYCLING

Technique

Make certain the seat height is correct for you and that you have comfortable padding on the seat for long rides. Adjust the handle bars to a position which is comfortable for your riding style. Pedaling must be vigorous and sustained to achieve real benefits, but relax and enjoy the sights!

Procedure

1. Start with a moderate pace so your leg muscles can adjust gradually to the increased activity.
2. Remember, it takes skill to safely handle a bike in traffic, on narrow roadways, and in tight situations. Learn how to handle your bike effectively before you attempt difficult situations such as heavy traffic or steep, winding roads. Be alert to holes or debris on the road.
3. Generally, you need to cycle twice as fast as you would jog to achieve your target heart rate (4). In the beginning strive for a sustained ride and gradually increase your time or distance.

Suggested Program   Under 30 years of age (2)

Week	Frequency (Per Week)	Distance (miles)	Time (min.)
1	3	2.0	9:00
2	3	2.0	8:00
3	3	3.0	10:45
4	4	3.0	10:00
5	4	4.0	15:00
6	4	4.0	14:30
7	4	5.0	18:30
8	4	5.0	18:00
9	5	5.0	27:30
10	4	6.0	22:30
11	4	6.0	22:00
12	4	6.0	21:30

AQUA DYNAMICS

Technique

Use these activities to improve cardiovascular endurance and to increase muscle tone, flexibility, calorie burn-up, and release of tensions. These activities are for the swimmer or non-swimmer. If possible, stay in water that is at shoulder level — the resistance of the water increases the strenuousness of your workout.

Procedure

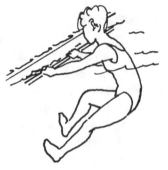

1. Choose a variety of strokes and make your workout continuous. Change strokes as you need to. See the suggested starter program which follows.
2. Select a variety of exercises and perform them in a sequence that will keep your heart rate in the target zone.
3. Consider having music available and combining many of your aerobic dance steps with the usual water exercises.

Suggested Program   Under 30 years of age (2)

Swimming Program (overhand crawl)

Week	Frequency (Per Week)	Distance (yards)	Time (min.)
1	4	300	12:00
2	4	300	10:30
3	4	300	10:15
4	5	500	20:00
5	5	500	18:00
6	5	500	17:00
7	5	200	4:00
8	5	300	6:00
9	5	400	8:30
10	5	500	10:30
11	5	600	12:30
12	4	800	15:30

WATER EXERCISE PROGRAM

Warm-up Exercises

Quadriceps Stretch
(Improves quadriceps flexibility)

While standing, bring the heel to the buttocks, grasping the top of the right foot with the right hand and pulling the heel towards the buttocks. Slowly, release and repeat with the left leg. (Hold onto the edge of the pool if necessary.)
   Note: Do not pull the knee out to the side.

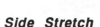

Side Stretch
(Heel cord, calf flexibility

Take a large stride forward, bending the right leg; keep the rear left leg straight, with the heel on the floor. Straighten the forward leg; relax and stretch. Keep both feet forward. Repeat with the other leg.

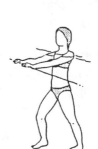

Upper Body Exercises

Lateral Arm Raises
(Shoulder and upper back)

With feet shoulder-width apart, arms to the side at shoulder-height and palms facing downward, cup the hands and pull arms down to the side. Turn palms up and pull arms back up to the starting position.

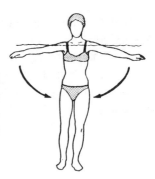

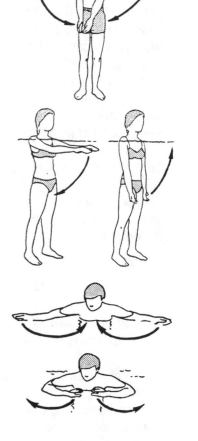

Horizontal Abduction/Adduction
(Chest and anterior shoulder)

Start with feet shoulder-width apart, arms at shoulder-height and to the sides, palms facing forward. Pull the arms together, and turn the palms out. Push to the starting position.

    Variation: Pull the arms across the body in a V-shape. Push the arms up at the same angle.

Shoulder Flexion/Extension
(Shoulders)

With feet shoulder-width apart, arms straight at shoulder-height in front of the body, palms facing down, pull the arms to the thighs, turning the palms up and pulling up to shoulder-height. Repeat.

Triceps-Biceps
(Upper Arms)

With feet shoulder-width apart, begin with the arms extended out to the sides at shoulder-height, palms facing forward. Bend the elbows and touch the hands to the chest; straighten the arms with the palms facing forward away from the chest.

Arm Raise
(Shoulder and chest)

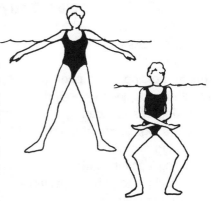

Stand in shoulder-deep water, legs shoulder-width apart, knees slightly bent. Raise arms to your sides, parallel to surface of water. Keep arms straight and palms facing toward pool bottom. Pull arms down in front of torso, then raise them to starting position, pushing against water. Repeat.

Training tip: Keep your arms underwater so you work against the resistance of the water throughout the exercise.

Lower Arm Paddling
(Front and back of upper arm)

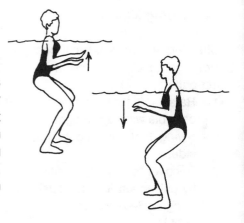

Stand in shoulder-deep water, legs shoulder-width apart, knees slightly bent. Begin with arms straight down at sides, palms upward. Keeping elbows in to your sides, raise lower arms. Turning hands so palms face pool bottom, straighten arms by pushing down. Turn hands so palms face upward. Repeat.

Lower Body Exercises

Leg Crosses

Supine, holding on to pool gutter with hands, legs extended:
1. Swing legs far apart.
2. Bring legs together crossing left leg over right.
3. Swing legs far apart.
4. Bring legs together crossing right leg over left. Repeat.

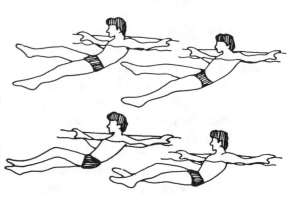

Leg Swing Outward

Standing with back against pool side and hands sideward, holding gutter:
1. Raise left foot as high as possible with leg straight.
2. Swing foot and leg to left side.
3. Recover to starting position by pulling left leg vigorously to right. Repeat. Reverse to right leg. Repeat.

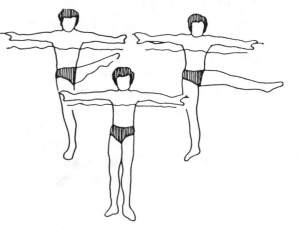

Back Flutter Kicking

Lying in a supine position and holding on to one side of pool with hand(s):
1. Flutter kick.

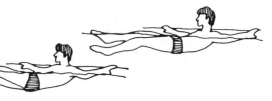

Front Flutter Kicking

Lying in a prone position holding on to side of pool with
hand(s):
1. Kick flutter style in which
   toes are pointed back, ankles are flexible, knee joint is
   loose but straight, and the
   whole leg acts as a whip.

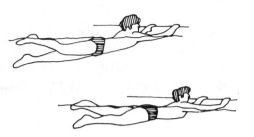

Knees Up Twisting

Supine, holding on to pool gutter with knees drawn up to
chest:
1. Twist slowly to left; recover
2. Twist slowly to right; recover
4. Repeat.

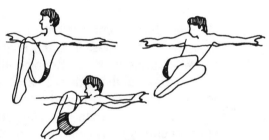

Kickboard Exercises

Waist Twists
(Shoulders and waist)

Standing with shoulder-width apart and
knees bent, hold the board lengthwise
at 90° and submerge it halfway into the
water. Move the board right to left,
keeping the hips facing forward. Movement is from the waist. Keep your eyes
on the board while twisting.

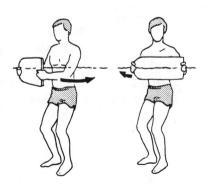

Pushups with Board
(Triceps)

Hold the board lengthwise (flat), with the arms bent and elbows extended out at the sides. Then, push the board down, straightening the arms as you go. Relax, and repeat.

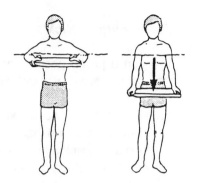

Tricep Push with Board
(Upper arms)

With the elbows bent straight in front and close to the sides, hold the board lengthwise at the surface. Keeping the elbows close to the sides, push the board down and bring it to the thighs, straightening the arms as you go. Return to starting position, and repeat. You may also place the hands on top of the board and push down.

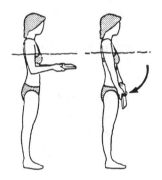

Bench Press
(Chest and upper back)
Hold the board perpendicular, and submerge it halfway under the water. Push forward and pull backwards as fast as possible.

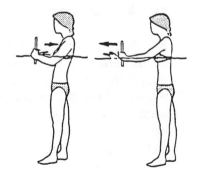

Cardiovascular Exercises

Hop and Turn

Standing upright, hop/jump as high as possible turning left or right. Absorb the shock of landing by bending the knees. Follow through by landing on the toes and rolling onto the balls and then the heels of the feet.

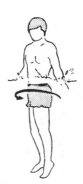

Side Straddle Hop

Standing in waist to chest-deep water with hands hips:
1. Jump sideward to position with feet approximately two feet apart.
2. Recover

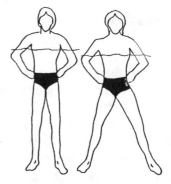

Jumping

With arms at your side and legs together, jump straight up. Land with knees bent.

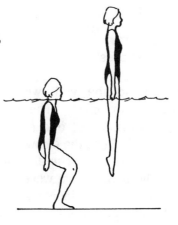

Stride Hop

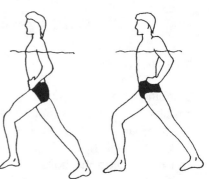

Stand in waist to chest-deep water with hands on hips:
1. Jump with left leg forward and right leg back.
2. Jump changing to right leg forward and left leg back.
   Repeat.

Wall Exercises

Wall Pushups I
(Triceps)

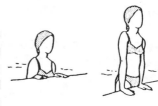

Stand facing the pool wall with the hands on top of the edge. Fingers pointing forward and the hands shoulder-with apart, keep the body rigid and extend upward. Then, press downwards with the arms, lifting the body out of the water without the assistance of the legs.

Variation: Face the fingers toward each other.

Wall Pushups II
(Triceps and chest)

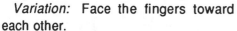

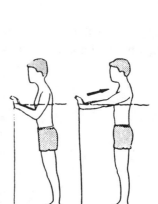

Stand facing the wall with hands shoulder-width apart. The legs are straight with the feet one to two feet from the wall. Bend the elbows, and the straighten the arms. The arms accommodate the body weight while performing the pushups. To increase difficulty, stand further from the wall.

Wall Sit Up
(Stomach)

Rest calves on the pool deck. With arms crossed on the chest, slowly curl upward. Hold ten seconds when shoulders are out of the water.

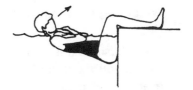

WORKOUT SCHEDULE FOR WATER EXERCISES

Weeks 1-2

Frequency: Three time a week with a rest day between workouts.

Intensity: Work at a speed that lets you feel the resistance of the water. Maintain control and correct form, particularly when learning the exercise.

Duration: 2 sets of 20 repetitions for each exercise. For exercises that use the right and left sides of the body separately, one set consists of 20 repetitions with each side.

Weeks 3-4

Frequency: Do exercises five days a week with two nonconsecutive rest days.

Intensity: Increase cadence of each repetition slightly over that of weeks 1-2. Maintain control and correct form.

Duration: 3 sets of 20 repetitions. For exercises that use the right and left sides of the body separately, one set consists of 20 repetitions with each side.

Weeks 5-6

Frequency: Six days a week.

Intensity: Increase speed of movement slightly over that of weeks 3-4. Maintain control and correct form.

Duration: 4 sets of 20 repetitions. For exercises that use the right and left sides of the body separately, one set consists of 20 repetitions with each side.

QUESTIONS AND ANSWERS

Which type of exercise will help me burn up the most calories?

The basic rule is that the fuel you burn is governed by the amount of weight you move and the distance you move it. Therefore, the same exercises which contribute to cardiovascular fitness are those which burn the most calories. Select activities which involve total body activity, which are rhythmical, and which can be maintained for a longer time. Aerobic dancing is great!

What is the best way to breathe when I jog?

The main way is to breathe normally and respond naturally to the increased demands on the body. For maximum ventilation, breathe in and out through both mouth and nose. In addition, it will help to relax and feel more comfortable if you periodically and forcibly exhale through the mouth.

Should I take salt tablets?

Contrary to what many people have thought, it is not necessary to increase your intake of salt when exercising during hot weather. Not only do we get enough salt in our normal diets, but the body learns to conserve salt so we are not losing as much as previously believed. Studies now show that sweat is mostly water.

Does exercising cause problems for women by displacing the uterus or stretching the ligaments in the breasts (causing them to droop)?

There is no evidence to support these fears. Actually, most doctors encourage women to exercise. Women in top physical condition generally have less menstrual discomfort, fewer backaches, fewer colds, less digestive disorders, and less fatigue than women who do not exercise. Women who exercise report greater firmness of the breasts due to loss of body fat and improved tone of the pectoral muscles. Displacement of the uterus is extremely unlikely since it has one of the best shock-absorbing systems in the human body (1).

Is exercising during pregnancy unsafe?

Most physicians indicate that if women were exercising before pregnancy, there is no reason they cannot continue during pregnancy. Of course, it is advisable to consult with your doctor to determine the exact exercise program for you. It may be necessary to make certain adjustments in your program from time to time. For a more complete discussion, see Chapter 8.

SUGGESTED LABS

Lab 12 — Blood Pressure
Lab 13 — RISKO

REFERENCES

1. Getchell, Bud. *The Fitness Book.* Benchmark Press Inc., Indianapolis, IN, 1987.
2. YMCA. *Physical Fitness Through Water Exercise.* National Board of YMCA, Rosemont, Illinois, 1982.
3. Knopf, Fleck, and Martin. *Water Workouts.* Hunter Textbooks Inc., Winston-Salem, NC, 1988.

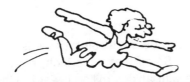

Chapter Six

Catch Your Beat
AEROBIC DANCE

For more than a decade aerobic dance has been one of the most popular forms of exercise. According to Dr. Richie, a sportsmedicine podiatrist, more than 22 million people are currently involved in aerobic dance programs (8). Because of the widespread popularity and the media attention which has accompanied its success, aerobic dance has become a household word.

Aerobic dance is a combination of different forms of dance, including disco, jazz and folk. The choreography is set to music which motivates and creates an atmosphere of energy and camaraderie unlike any other exercise class. The physiological, psychological and sociological benefits of aerobic dance can have a very positive effect on the quality of your life. Before beginning your aerobic dance program, there are some guidelines you should follow.

GET READY
Shoes

In an aerobic dance class, you should always wear shoes specifically designed for aerobic dance. Running and other sports shoes are inappropriate. Aerobic dance shoes have two basic functions. First, the shoe is made to protect and stabilize the foot while helping to absorb the shock of impact that occurs during the workout. The shoe is designed to accommodate the horizontal, lateral, and vertical movements characteristic of aerobic dance. The second function of the shoe is to help protect the feet from undesirable floor surfaces. The shock absorbent qualities of an aerobic shoe become critical when the floor surface is non-shock absorbing, such as concrete. A good aerobic dance floor, together with a good aerobic shoe, significantly reduces the shock of impact created when your foot meets the floor.

Choosing a good aerobic shoe can be a difficult task. It is helpful to begin by determining foot shape. Some feet have high, rigid arches, while others are flat and unstable with ankles rolling inward. Once you have determined your foot shape, it becomes easier to select the right type of shoe. When selecting a shoe, traction, stability, flexibility and cushioning are important considerations. Recent studies indicate that the midsole of the shoe is important for absorbing about 60 percent of impact shock. To test mid-sole stability, twist the shoe at the heel and toe and if it can be easily twisted, it will probably not provide adequate stability. Shoes should fit snugly, have a slightly elevated sole and provide adequate lateral support. It is also a good idea to wear socks to prevent blisters.

Shoes for aerobic dance should be tested for flexibility and cushioning. Look for a slightly elevated heel.

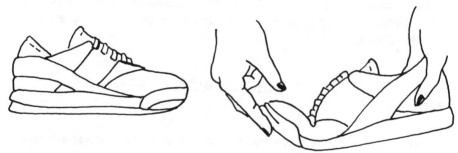

Clothing

Aerobic dance attire should be loose fitting and made of a porous material like cotton to insure maximum comfort and easy movement. Tights and leotards help keep the body temperature at optimum level for exercise. Warm-up suits made of plastic, rubber and other non-porous materials should be avoided. They can lead to dehydration, decreased work capacity and various forms of heat illnessess. The loss of body weight immediately following aerobics while wearing such a suit is only water and lasts until fluids are ingested.

Excessive breast movement during aerobic dance class can be a problem for some women, especially those with large breasts. The discomfort is usually caused by an inadequate intrinsic support system, and can be minimized or eliminated by using a sports bra. The best way for a woman to judge a bra is to try it on and jog in place. Some features of a quality sports bra Include:

1. Fabric made of at least 50 percent cotton, to minimize chafing
2. Covered hooks
3. Rear closure
4. Non-elastic shoulder straps
5. A cup-type support made of non-elastic material

GET SET

After assessing your present fitness level, establishing guidelines for the exercise prescription, and completing Labs 1 and 2 of this text, you are ready to begin your aerobic dance program. Medical clearance is especially important for the elderly, the obese and those with a history of heart disease. If you have any questions about your medical status, consult your physician before beginning your aerobic dance program.

In your aerobic program, you will apply the Frequency, Intensity, and Time (FIT) principle. Except for poorly-conditioned individuals, exercise should be done at least three times per week to produce a measurable training effect. It is more desirable to increase the time of the activity than to increase the intensity. Research has documented that you must exercise at an intensity equal to 60 percent of your maximum heart rate. Except in the case of world-class athletes, training at an intensity greater than 85 percent is not necessary and may in fact be counterproductive. To determine your target heart rate, refer to the information in Chapters 3 and 4.

Guidelines for Aerobic Exercise

Training Level	Days Per Week	Frequency Minutes	Intensity % of Maximal HeartRate
Beginning	3	20	60%
Intermediate	4	30	75%
Advanced	5-6	45	80-85%

As you begin your exercise program, start slowly and do not work too hard too soon. Initially, workouts should be at a low intensity to allow the body to gradually adapt to the exercise program. Injuries and discomfort occur too frequently when one begins at a high level of intensity. Low intensity/longer duration is preferable to high intensity/short duration. The interaction between intensity and duration should be such that you do not experience undue fatigue after the exercise session.

Progress in your aerobic dance program is dependent on your fitness level, age, health, and goals that you set for yourself. As you progress in your program, you should gradually increase the intensity of your workout. It will take between 4-6 weeks before results will become evident.

GO

A well-organized, smooth flowing aerobic dance class will generally consist of five segments, although individual teaching styles may have variations of the following sequences:

* Warmup exercises including light calisthenics: 10 minutes

The warm-up prepares the cardiovascular system for the aerobic workout, by increasing the body's core temperature and the flow of blood to all the working muscles. The warm-up should include static stretching and rhythmic, light calisthenics. Arm swings, knee raises, and small kicks are examples of rhythmic, warm-up activities.

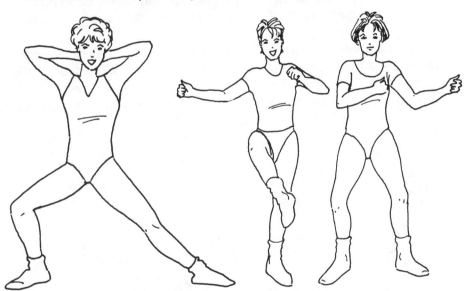

Side-lunge
Legs are turned out with the knees placed directly over the toes. The arms are placed comfortably behind the head, elbows back. Lunge side to side, shifting the weight evenly between both legs. Repeat and then hold the lunge position each side for ten seconds.

Rhythmic Limbering
Step-kick low and with control. Use the arms in a side-to-side motion to warm the upper body. Coordinate both the arms and legs with smooth, controlled movement.

* Aerobic Activity: 15-60 minutes
(varies with fitness level)

The aerobic segment consists of rhythmic, large muscle exercises that can be sustained for a predetermined amount of time. High leg lifts, step-touch movements, high kicks, and controlled lunges are examples of such exercises. These kinds of aerobic movements will cause the heart and respiratory rates to increase which enhances the flow of oxygen to the muscles.

The tempo of the music and the range of movement gradually increase resulting in a greater workload for the heart and lungs. This increase is important because unless the exercise becomes more demanding, there is no aerobic training effect. The minimum intensity should be 60 percent of maximum heart rate and the maximum should not exceed 85 percent.

At various intervals during the aerobic segment, heart rates should be monitored. The pulse should be taken at either the radial (wrist) or carotid (neck) artery. For the most accurate reading, use your forefinger and middle finger to detect the pulse. Taking an accurate pulse may require some practice before it is perfected.

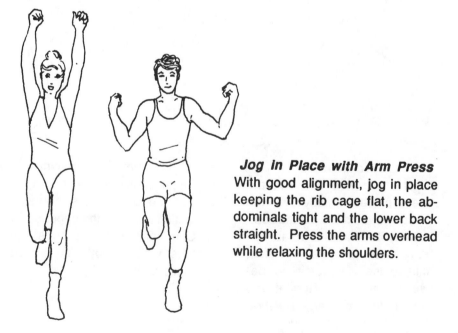

Jog in Place with Arm Press
With good alignment, jog in place keeping the rib cage flat, the abdominals tight and the lower back straight. Press the arms overhead while relaxing the shoulders.

Scissors Stepping

Alternate feet in a lunge position, using opposite arms with legs. Press the heels into the floor when landing. Keep the body aligned with the knees over the toes.

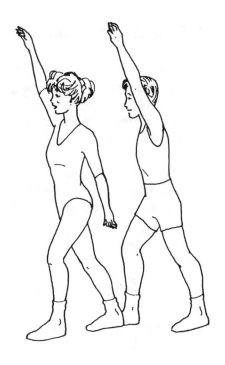

High Kicks

Lift the leg, keeping the torso straight and properly aligned. The heel should be pressed into the floor with each landing

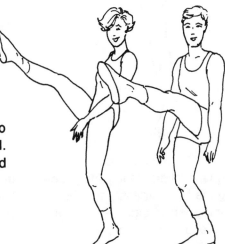

* Post Aerobic Cool-down: 8 minutes

The intensity of an aerobic workout should end gradually so as to allow the muscles to assist in pumping blood from the extremities back to the heart. An abrupt stop in exercise can result in blood pooling in the lower extremities which may cause a drop in blood pressure leading to nausea, dizziness or fainting.

During the cool-down period, the heart rate should be less than 60 percent of maximum. This can be accomplished by walking and repeating some of the exercises used during the warm-up segment.

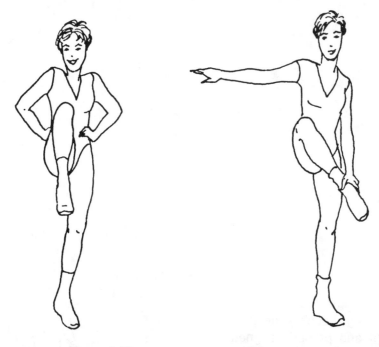

Knee Lift	*Alternate Heel Touch*
In place, alternate leg lifting, keeping the back straight, and the supporting leg straight. Relax shoulders and breathe deeply.	In place, touch opposite hand to heel of the foot. Keep the back straight and the abdominal muscles tight. Repeat.

* Exercises for muscular strength and endurance: 20 minutes

Depending on the length of the class, the muscular endurance section can last from 20-45 minutes. At this time, the abdominal, adductor, abductor and gluteal muscles can be exercised specifically. Proper breathing techniques, proper alignment and the concept of controlled movements are important aspects of this section. The use of rubber bands or light weights can be added for the intermediate and advanced student.

Abdominal Crunch with Twist
Press the abdominals into the floor. Reach across the body while relaxing the neck and shoulders. Repeat.

Reverse Sit-ups
Lift the knees to the chest, raising the hips off the floor. Do not let the knees go past the shoulders. Roll back to the floor, slowly and carefully. Repeat.

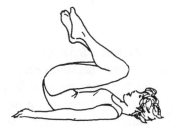

Leg Extension
Place the upper body on the floor. Extend the leg slowly upward keeping it in line with the torso. Lower your leg slowly and repeat with the other side.

* Final Stretch: 5 minutes

The major focus of the final stretch is relaxation. All of the muscles used in the workout should be statically stretched with particular emphasis on the calf, hamstrings, and back. This part of class is helpful for improving flexibility. Being flexible greatly reduces the chances of injury during rigorous aerobic activity.

Hamstring and Lower Back Stretch

Extend one leg, keeping the hips square. Bend the other leg in towards the body. Gently press the body forward leading from the hips until a slight tension is felt. Hold the stretch for 30 seconds. Relax and repeat on the other side.

Straddle Stretch

Place both hips squarely on the floor. Stretch forward from the hips and place the body on the leg. Alternate the positions as illustrated. Repeat each side two times.

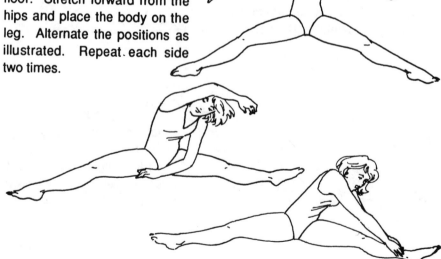

ALIGNMENT FOR MOVEMENT

Good body alignment is important for all phases of the aerobic workout. By keeping body parts in a properly aligned position, you will reduce the chances of sustaining an injury and at the same time improve your balance, coordination and agility.

The term *alignment* refers to a balanced posture while standing, sitting, or lying down. The proper alignment in the standing position is described as the trunk being held in a neutral position. From this neutral position, the rest of the body should be aligned in the following ways:

1. The head should be held on top of the spine, straightforward with the chin in line with the chest. If the head is held in front of or in back of the spine, there will be unnecessary shoulder and neck tension.

2. The shoulders should appear square on the body and remain relaxed.

3. The pelvis and the hips should be neutral avoiding a forward or backward tilt which might cause a hyperextended lower back.

4. The knees should be aligned with the feet and be placed directly over the feet when landing from a jump. The knees should be flexed on impact to help dissipate shock.

5. The feet should distribute the weight of the body from toe-to-heel with the heel of the foot coming all the way down to the floor. Pressing the heels to the floor is a significant factor in minimizing shin splints.

BODY ALIGNMENT

Three Views for Proper Body Alignment

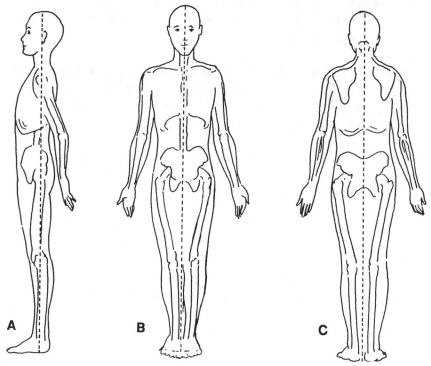

Normal postural alignment: A, Side view; **B,** Front view; **C,** Back view

Proper Alignment for Sitting And Standing

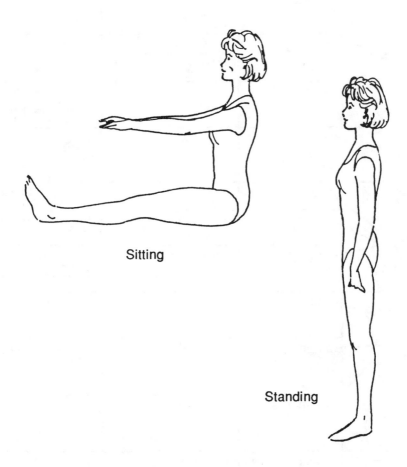

Sitting

Standing

To achieve good alignment, it is helpful to visualize the relationship of body parts, one to another and to do a posture analysis (Lab 14). Becoming familiar with good alignment and body mechanics requires practice and concentration but it is necessary for an injury-free aerobic dance experience.

TABLE 1
ANATOMICAL AWARENESS

PART OF BODY	MAIN MUSCLES	APPROXIMATE LOCATION	MAIN MOVEMENT
ARMS AND SHOULDER	TRICEPS	Bottom of upper arm (when arm is lifted to side at right angle to body with palm up)	Straightens or extends elbow
	BICEPS	Top of upper arm (when arm is lifted to side at right angle to body with palm up)	Bends or flexes elbow
	PECTORALS	Front of chest	Rotate arm inward in shoulder socket and control some other arm movements
	TRAPEZIUS AND OTHER MUSCLES OF THE UPPER BACK	Upper back	Move scapulae (shoulder blades)
ABDOMEN	OBLIQUES	Over ribs on either side	Twists upper body to either side
	RECTUS ABDOMINIS	From upper ribs to top of pubic bone, covering abdomen area	Raises upper body forward as in sit-up
	QUADRATUS LUMBORUM	Small of back	1. Bends upper body to side 2. Stabilizes pelvis and spine
HIP AND UPPER LEG (THIGH)	GLUTEALS	Buttocks	1. Stabilize hip 2. Extend hip
	QUADRICEPS	Front of thigh	Extends leg in forward movements
	HAMSTRINGS	Back of upper leg	Bend knee
LOWER LEG	GASTROCNEMIUS (GASTROX OR CALF)	Back of lower leg	1. Points foot 2. *Raises* leg to ball of foot (half toe) 3. Bends knee
	SOLEUS	Back of lower leg under gastrox muscle	*Holds* leg in half-toe position (ball of foot)
	TIBIALIS AND PERONEUS	Around either side of ankle	Move ankle in circle
	ACHILLES TENDON	Lower part of leg and heel on back of leg; lower part of gastrox (calf) muscle	Same as gastrox

Adapted from *The Dancer Prepares: Modern Dance for Beginners,* 2e by James Penrodd and Janice Gudde Plastino by permission of Mayfield Publishing Company. Copyright © by Mayfield Publishing Company.

AEROBIC DANCE INJURIES

Even with good alignment and good instruction, there is always a possibility of injury while participating in aerobic dance. Aerobic dance, like other activities, combines lateral, horizontal, and vertical movements which can lead to injuries. While providing an enjoyable way to fitness, there have been a significant number of musculoskeletal injuries resulting from aerobic dance. The majority of these are from overuse and occur primarily in the lower leg (shin), foot, and ankle. Some of the reasons cited for these injuries include:

1. Increased hours of participation
2. Improper footwear
3. Non-resilient floor surfaces

Some of the more common dance injuries include the following:

Plantar fasciitis is an inflammation of the plantar fascia, a tendon-like structure which lies in the arch and metatarsal area of the foot. It may become strained, irritated or torn if enough stress or repetitive action is applied. A high-arched foot and tight Achilles tendon predispose this condition.

The treatment for plantar fasciitis includes rest, anti-inflammatory medication, and proper shoe selection. Therapeutic options for the treatment of plantar fasciitis include shoe orthotics to correct foot imbalances, ice massage and stretching exercises.

Shin splints is a condition characterized by pain in the middle or outer part of the front of the lower leg. In most cases, shin splints is caused by overtraining, inadequate floor surfaces, improper shoes and improper instruction. In some specific cases, the cause may be attributed to stress fractures, muscle strains, tendonitis, and compartment syndrome, which is a severe condition of shin splints.

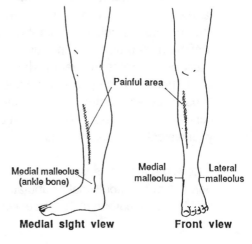

Painful area

Medial malleolus (ankle bone)

Medial malleolus

Lateral malleolus

Medial sight view

Front view

The best treatment for shin splints is prevention. Your chances of experiencing this common aerobic dance injury will be reduced if you select a good pair of shoes, and dance on a quality floor surface. Orthotics may be helpful, especially for those who suffer from chronic foot problems. Treatment for shin splints consists of ice massage, stretching and rest. In severe cases anti-inflammatory drug therapy may be necessary.

Whenever an injury occurs during aerobic exercise, you should get a professional evaluation and follow-up treatment. It is not recommended that you return to activity before your injury has been treated and rehabilitated.

Stress Fracture is a hairline break in a bone usually occurring in the weight-bearing locations of the body, such as the foot and lower leg (tibia). Stress fractures occur gradually with an accompanying pain over the injured area. The condition is progressive and usually becomes worse if weight- bearing activities continue. If the injury is unattended, a complete fracture may occur.

The treatment of a stress fracture consists of applying ice for 20-30 minutes after activity or when there is pain. All weight-bearing activities, such as running and jumping, should be avoided until the symptoms have disappeared. Exercise intensity should then be increased very gradually.

Chondromalacia is a degenerative condition in which the back surface of the kneecap becomes softer and rougher. The exact cause of the condition is unknown, but it is suspected that body mechanics, foot pronation, and abnormal position of the knee may contribute to it. This injury occurs more frequently with girls and women because of the angle of the pelvis, which places the kneecap in a more outward position and causes rubbing of the undersurface of the knee. The treatment for this condition is ice massage for 2-3 minutes after exercise and a decrease in your weight-bearing activities.

Low back pain is very common in the United States. More than 50 percent of the adult male population each year will suffer from a back problem and more than 80 percent of these will be muscle related. Some of the most frequent causes of low back discomfort are poor posture, improper body mechanics, lack of flexibility, and weak abdominals. Quick lateral or twisting movements of the trunk or hyperextension of the back can cause chronic pain and/or a sharp stabbing sensation.

General Rules for First Aid

A general rule to follow when an injury occurs in class is the RICE principle: rest, Ice, compression, and elevation. Rest is important because it eliminates further injury to the injured joint or muscle. Ice is applied for the first 24 to 48 hours to reduce swelling. Compression is helpful in preventing any additional swelling as is elevation which uses the effect of gravity. And finally, if the injury becomes chronic, ice should be applied when the swelling occurs and the participant should consult a physician.

LOW-IMPACT AEROBIC DANCE — LIAD

In response to the increasing number of injuries sustained in aerobic dance classes, an alternative form of dance exercise referred to as "low impact" aerobic dance was started. Low impact differs from high impact in that one foot is always on the floor throughout the aerobic segment of the workout. There are more upper body movements combined with low kicks, high stepping, and controlled lunges. By eliminating the repetitive effect of high impact aerobics, there is less stress on the joints and less chance of incurring overuse injuries or shin splints.

Low impact aerobic dance is becoming even more popular than its counterpart, high impact. Because of the different approach to the workout, the sedentary, the overweight and the elderly can participate without the high risk of injury or embarrassment. Low impact classes are also recommended for people with alignment problems, a history of previous injuries, and foot deformities.

By adding light hand or wrist weights, low impact workouts can be a challenge for the intermediate and advanced student. The weights, when used properly can help elevate the heart rate to the target zone. The weights should be between 1/2 and 2 pounds and should be used with some caution. Good technique and instruction on how to use the weights properly is very important. Improper use of the weights can cause tendonitis of the elbow or wrist. The use of ankle weights in an aerobic class can cause stress fractures and Achilles tendon problems and, therefore, should be avoided.

Most studies indicate that low impact aerobics meet the criteria for aerobic training as outlined by the American College of Sports Medicine. Low intensity classes can burn fat as effectively as higher intensity if the exercise is done long enough. In addition to being as effective as high impact aerobics, low impact is as much fun and as much a challenge as high impact aerobic dance. The effectiveness of the class depends on the fitness level of the participant and the ability of the instructor to teach the class safely.

Low-impact Aerobic Dance Exercises

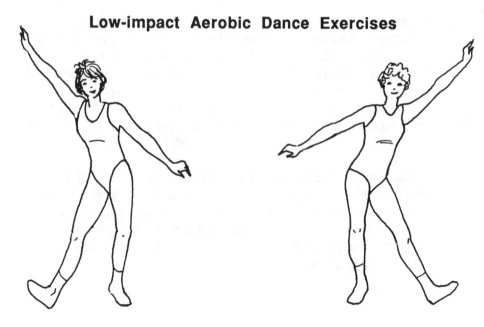

Heel Touch
Keeping one foot on the floor, touch heel to floor, alternate sides and use arms to increase the intensity of the movement.

Twists

Jump with feet together, knees flexed and arms moving up and down. Maintain body alignment and avoid arching the back.

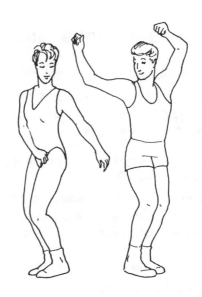

Forward Lunge with Arm Press

Knees are slightly flexed, step forward with one foot, remembering to bend the knee, so that it is perpendicular to the floor. At the same time extend the arms forward with control and good form. Alternate the legs using the same arm and leg and then alternating sides.

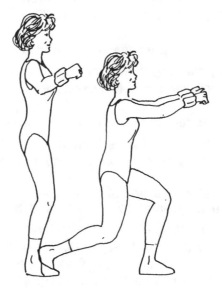

QUESTIONS AND ANSWERS

Will doing aerobic activity get rid of cellulite?

Cellulite does not exist. There is one type of fat and all fat must be treated in the same way in an exercise program. Special machines, pills, and diets for cellulite are useless.

If I work out aerobically three times a week, will I definitely lose weight?

Do not expect to lose weight if you do not watch your diet. You may lose fat while seeming to stay the same weight on the scale. A pound of muscle does not take up the same space as a pound of fat.

When is the best time of the day to exercise?

Exercising before breakfast may lead to more rapid weight loss than exercising before dinner. According to the results of a study done comparing morning and evening exercises, morning exercisers had 25 percent greater weight loss.

What is the purpose of wearing leg warmers?

They may help to keep the muscles of the legs warm although there is no scientific evidence to support this.

Is it better to eat before or after aerobic dance class?

This is a personal decision which must be determined by you. However, most individuals prefer eating *after* aerobic activity.

How effective are machines and devices that are electrically driven in promoting fitness and burning calories?

Not effective at all. The cliche "You only get out of something what you put into it" says it all. To burn calories and increase fitness levels, your muscles must work; the harder muscles work, the greater involvement there is for the circulatory system, respiratory system and other body functions.

Will exercise make me live longer?

Although there is no guarantee that exercise will add years to your life, there is no question that it will add life to your years. You basically inherit your capacity for longevity. However, a very comprehensive long term study, investigating the effect of lifestyle on mortality, has indicated that exercising enough to burn 2000 calories per week can reduce the chances of dying of a heart attack by 64 percent.

How effective are body wrapping and wearing sauna pants for effectively reducing body fat?

They are gimmicks. People are led to believe they have lost weight with such methods because of the before and after measurements. The loss of weight is simply a loss of body fluids. These techniques not only do nothing to remove body fat effectively, but they can also be hazardous to people with circulatory problems.

Can exercise increase breast size?

No. Breasts are primarily fat tissue which is not affected by exercise. In fact, the lack of exercise when it leads to an increase in weight, can cause breast size to increase. An effective weight training program can develop the pectoral (chest) muscles and increase the circumference of the chest, but the cup size will remain the same.

Is it harmful to exercise while menstruating?

In most cases, no. Painful breasts are a common problem for some females with most of the swelling caused by water retention. Olympic records have been set by women during their menstrual cycle. If you are one of the many women who sometimes get cramps or low back pain on the first or second day of your period, try exercising. The increase in blood flow to the pelvis may ease the discomfort by releasing the tension which is a contributing factor to cramps. Unless you have extremely severe or unusual problems, do not use your period as an excuse not to exercise. You may be missing out on the very thing that can ease the discomfort.

What are the characteristics of a quality aerobic dance class?

When selecting an aerobic dance class, the most important consideration should be the qualifications of the instructor. A good teacher can make aerobic dance a fun and meaningful experience. Look for a professional who has experience and training in physicale ducation, dance or a health-related service. Persons without this training should have completed a certification program presented by an organization with credibility. The second most important characteristic of a quality program is the floor. A resilient floor is important in helping to minimize injuries.

What are the important qualities of an aerobic dance shoe?

A good pair of aerobic shoes protect and stabilize the foot while helping to absorb the shock of impact with the floor during aerobic exercise. Other important considerations include traction, flexibility, and cushioning. The shoes should fit snugly and have adequate lateral support with a slightly elevated sole.

Are low-impact aerobics as beneficial as high impact aerobics?

Low-impact aerobics is safer than high energy aerobics and provides similar cardiovascular benefits. A low-impact aerobic class incorporates more upper body movements and lateral activities without excessive strain on the muscles and joints of the body.

SUGGESTED LABS

Lab 14 — Posture Analysis
Lab 16 — Aerobic Dance Workout

REFERENCES

1. Campbell, M.K. and Ogard. M.A. "Lower Leg Injuries in Aerobic Dance." *Acute Care and Rehabilitation* 2 (10) 12, 1987.
2. Cooper, K.H. *The Aerobics Program for Total Well-Being*. Bantam Books, Toronto, 1982.
3. Hobson, A.J . and Robinson, J.P. *Aerobic Dance for Effective Performance*. Kendall /Hunt Publishing Co., Dubuque, IA,1987.
4. Koszulta, L.E. "Low-Impact Aerobics: Better Than Traditional Aerobic Dance." *The Physician and Sportsmedicine* 14 (7) : 156, 1986.
5. Legwood, G. " Does Aerobic Dance Offer More Fun Than Fitness?" *The Physician and Sportsmedicine* 10 (9): 156, 1982.
6. Nelson, D.J., Pelis, A.E., Greener, D.L. and White, T.P. "Cardiac Frequency and Caloric Cost of Aerobic Dance in Young Women." *Research Quarterly in Exercise and Sport* 59 (9) (3): 229, 1988.
7. Trapp, D.E. and Hollifield, N.L. *Aerobic Dance: A Focus on Fitness*. Burgess Publishing Co., Minneapolis, 1986.
8. Vetter, W.L. , Helfet, D.L., Spear, K. and Matthews, L. "Aerobic Dance Injuries." *The Physician and Sportsmedicine* 13 (2): 114, 1985.
9. Walsh, P.R. and Shephard, R.J. "Patellofemoral Arthralgia, Patellar Instability and Chrondomalacia Patella." *Current Therapy in Sportsmedicine.* Mosby Publishing Co., Toronto, 1986.
10. Wells, C.L. "Exercise Physiology," *Aerobic Dance-Exercise Instructor's Manual.* Idea Foundation, San Diego,1987
11. West, M.S. and Shelton, L. "Class Design and Conduct" *Aerobics: Theory and Practice.* HDL Communications, Costa Mesa, CA, 1988.

Chapter Seven

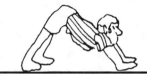

Get Physical
MUSCULAR FITNESS:
STRENGTH AND ENDURANCE

WHY?

Basic to any discussion of improving strength and endurance is an understanding of the value and benefits to be gained from the program. Many people, especially women, feel that since they are not interested in developing larger muscles (body building), there is no need for strength training. However, such an opinion overlooks the tremendous advantages of having an appropriate level of muscular strength and endurance.

There is ample evidence that stronger muscles better protect the joints which they cross, making you less prone to joint injuries. Muscles with greater strength and endurance are also less susceptible to strains, sprains, and pulls. Another important benefit is that better tone in the muscles of the trunk aids in preventing some of the common postural problems such as low back pain, round shoulders, and sagging abdominals. Additional reasons for maintaining an adequate level of strength and endurance are to enhance performance in sports, to lessen the effect of fatigue, to aid in the rehabilitation of injured muscles, and to help you look and feel better. As people improve their appearance by firming muscles and developing a better shape, their self-esteem and outlook on life usually improve.

In order to develop better strength fitness, each individual must first assess his or her particular level of strength and endurance. The selected tests in Chapter Two provide information about the areas in greatest need of improvement. Your specific goals will determine the type of exercise program which will produce the best results. Knowing the correct procedures for effective strength training will lead to faster improvement and fewer injuries.

Women are frequently concerned that they will develop large, bulky muscles by participating in weight training. Actually, the opposite occurs. A firm, well-contoured figure is usually found among women who participate in regular exercise of this kind. In addition, the potential for achieving muscle size and strength is largely determined by genetic makeup. This is why women usually do not develop large bulging muscles when involved in a weight training program. Females generally have about one-third fewer muscle fibers than men and it is the male hormone, testosterone, which contributes to muscle growth and hypertrophy. However, an individualized program for strength and muscular fitness can help women reach their optimal strength level.

HOW?

The basic ingredient of a muscular fitness training program is progressive resistance. The goal is to single out a specific muscle group and gradually apply greater and greater stress to it. A high intensity program (heavier weights or resistance) with fewer repetitions will specifically lead to gains in muscle strength. A low intensity (lighter weights or using one's body weight) with many repetitions (20 or more) will lead to gains in muscular endurance. In either program it is important to increase the intensity of the workout gradually so that the muscles will respond positively and not suffer extreme tissue damage. All of the principles and guidelines for training discussed in Chapter Three should be observed as one participates in a muscular fitness program.

1. **Natural Resistance** — your own body weight, manual resistance from a partner, and/or isometric exercises.

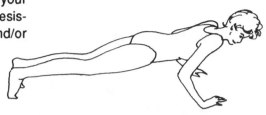

2. **Barbells and Dumbbells** — Commonly referred to as free weights, these can be utilized in a variety of ways. Barbells are designed for two-handed lifts and dumbbells for one-handed lifts. The amount of weight used may be varied and the equipment is relatively inexpensive.

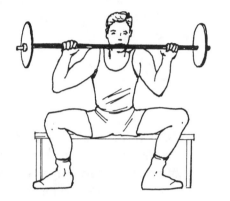

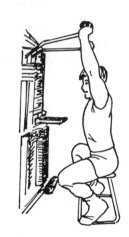

3. **Universal Gym Equipment** —This very popular weight training equipment has weight stacks which are lifted by lever and pulley attachments. The weights are on fixed tracks which make them safe, easily adjustable, and very convenient.

4. **Nautilus Equipment** — This equipment uses a cam system to provide resistance that changes to match the joint's ability to produce force throughout the range of motion and an accommodating resistance device.

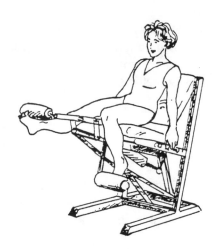

5. **Mini-Gym and Hydra-Gym Equipment**—Training devices that automatically vary the resistance in response to the amount of muscular force applied. This equipment enables one to perform exercises at a variety of speeds with maximum resistance.

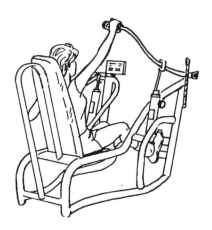

WHERE?

For individuals interested in learning more about the various types of weight training equipment and how to establish a specific program, it is best to investigate the publications listed below. These sources are very comprehensive and will give a more complete description of muscular strength and endurance.

Weight Training Everyone, Second Edition, by Tuten, Moore and Knight. Winston-Salem, NC: Hunter Textbooks Inc., 1986.

Strength Fitness: Physiological Principles and Training Techniques by Westcott. Boston: Allyn & Bacon, 1982.

Strength Training Principles by Darden. Winter Park, FL: Anna Publishing Co., 1977.

READY, SET, GO!

As previously stated, it is quite possible to develop muscular fitness by using the natural resistance of your body weight to help you. The following exercises are designed to be done at home or at school; all you need is a clear area of floor and possibly an exercise mat or padded carpet for comfort. Remember to warm up before starting and cool down when you finish. Start slowly with a few repetitions and increase the intensity as you progress. Many of these exercises are especially beneficial in improving muscular endurance.

ABDOMINALS

Basic Curl Up: Curl straight, twist to left, twist to right, and twist bringing opposite knee to elbow.

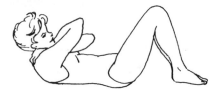

Curl up with arms extended to side of knees. Hold. Curl up with arms extended on outside of knees. Hold.

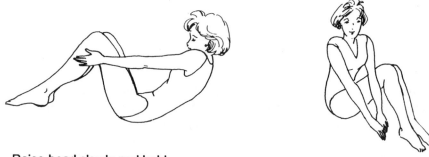

Raise head slowly and hold.

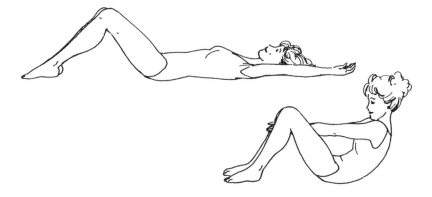

Elevated Leg Curls: Roll head, neck, and shoulders and hold.

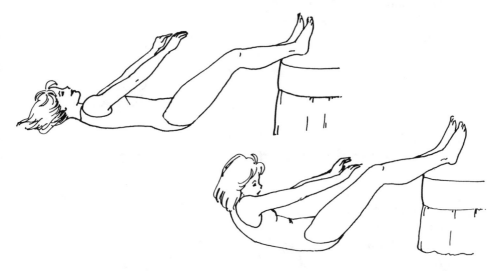

Sit-ups: Relax the neck and shoulders. Press lower abdominals into the floor as you lift the body.

16 ct. sit-ups — opposite elbow to the knee
16 ct. sit-ups — hands lightly placed on knees

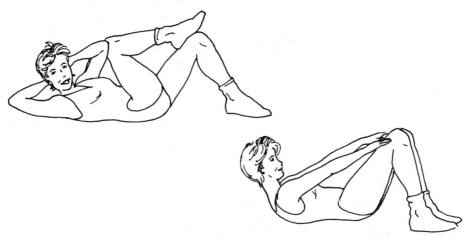

Press the lower back into the floor. Relax the neck and shoulders. Touch opposite elbow to knee.

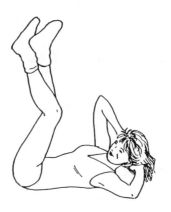

Beginning Abdominal Exercises

Hold weight on chest. Curl and twist opposite elbow toward raised knee. Keep other elbow on floor.

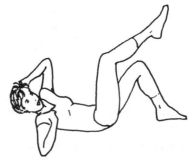

Rest weight on chest. Place both hands on forehead. Curl forward.

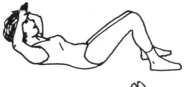

Place weight on chest. Curl toward legs, lifting pelvis off floor. Keep elbows back and chin up.

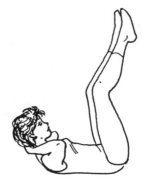

Advanced Abdominal Exercises

Keep knees bent and slowly pull legs up toward chin until buttocks are off the floor. Lower pelvis until buttocks touch floor.

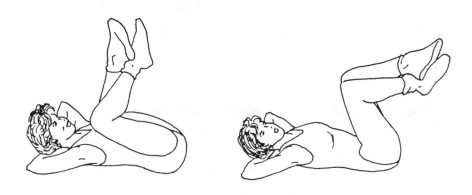

Raise head and shoulders as high as possible by bending at the waist. Keep body as straight as possible.

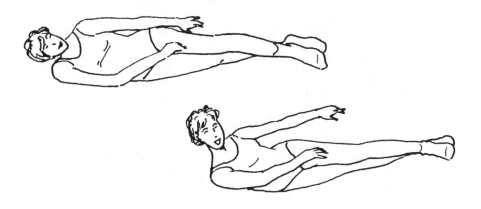

Triceps

Chair push-up

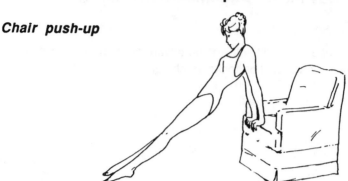

Tricep Press: Lift until arms are straight and hold. Lower slowly back to the floor.

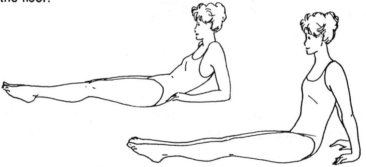

Quadriceps and Gluteals

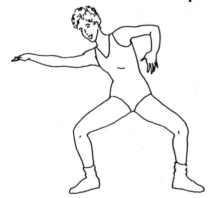

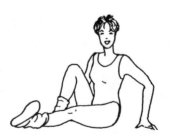

Knees over the toes. Shoulders over the hips. Abdominals tight and the back straight. Shoulders relaxed.

Back straight. Abdominals tight. Feet flexed. Lift slowly and carefully.

Thigh and Hip

Use ankle weights. Flex lower leg and raise it as high as possible toward ceiling. Hold. Slowly lower.

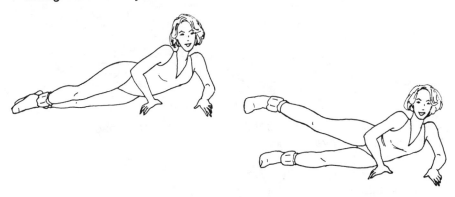

Use ankle weights. Bend bottom leg slightly. Extend upper leg with knee facing forward. Raise upper leg up toward ceiling with foot flexed. Hold. Slowly return to position.

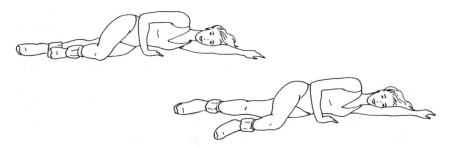

Raise extended leg and hold. Foot extended and then flexed.

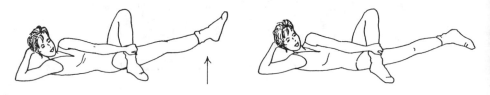

Use ankle weights. Tighten buttocks and bend one knee to lift leg slightly off ground. Slowly curl heel toward buttocks.

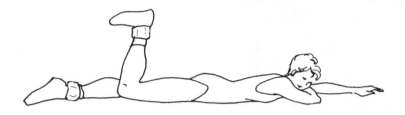

Use ankle weights. Raise straight leg no higher than back, tightening buttocks. Do not move torso or arch back.

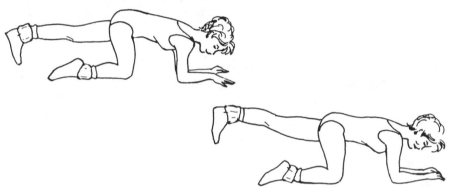

Use ankle weights. Lift one leg, keeping knee bent at 90° angle with ankle flexed and abdominals tightened. Tighten buttocks while lifting, then lower leg to ground. Keep head aligned with spine. Do not arch back or turn hip out.

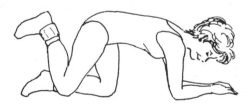

Use ankle weights. Bring one knee in to chest. Slowly extend leg straight back. Tighten buttocks at full extension. Do not arch back or raise hip.

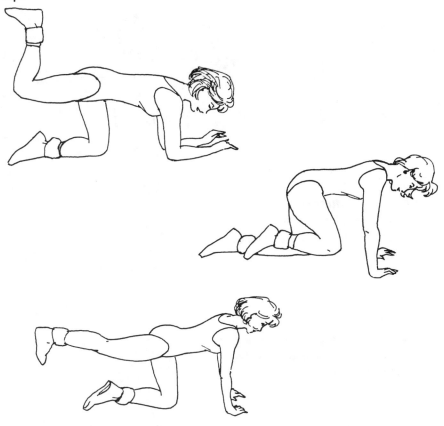

Pelvic Lift: Tighten abdominals and buttocks. Raise pelvis and hold. Lower slowly.

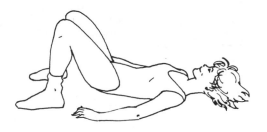

Partner Resistance

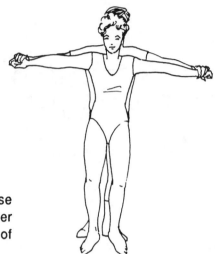

Shoulder Muscles: Raise arms to shoulder level as partner applies resistance to the back of the wrists.

Outside of Thigh: Raise leg as high as possible with resistance to side of leg.

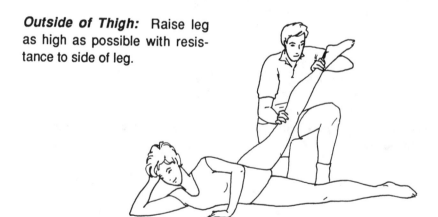

Shoulder: Raise arm as resistance is applied to back of hand.

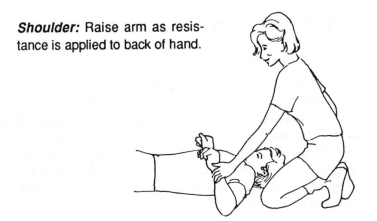

Hamstring Curl: Raise leg with toes pointed toward knee. Raise as high as possible, hold, and return slowly to ground. Resist at the heel and leg.

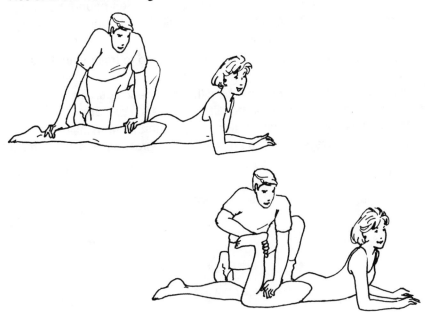

QUESTIONS AND ANSWERS

Are there differences in weight training?

When it comes to weight training, there is very little agreement. However, there are roughly three schools of thought on purpose. First, there is the pure "weight lifter," whose primary purpose is developing mass or bulk to see how much he or she can lift. Next, comes the "body builder," whose main purpose in life is to develop size and symmetry of muscles. Strength is not a prime concern here. Finally, we have the "weight trainer" whose interest is to develop endurance, size, strength and flexibility, with the end result being to enhance performance.

How much should I increase my "weight load" from week to week?

Since many weight machines increase their weights in increments of 10-15 and sometimes 20 pounds, this can present a problem. It is recommended that one increase the weight by no more than five percent each week; however, this may be less than the ten-pound increment. One must therefore be cautious and patient until the increased weight can be safely added. Remember that:

- Each person is different and does not respond to training in the same way.
- The entry level of strength will be different for each person.
- Maximum strength limits will be different for each person.
- Initial gains will be greater for those who are farther from their limit.
- Less gains always occur as an individual approaches his or her maximum limits.

As a female, I am not interested in gaining strength, but I would like to body build in a few spots. Any suggestions?

Assuming you are in good health, the following guidelines for training should be helpful:

• Remember to begin with light weights to practice the basic techniques.
• Do only one set of 10-12 reps per exercise.
• Work every other day for one or two weeks, then increase your workout to two sets.
• After one or two weeks increase your workout to three sets.
• The next step is to increase your weight and to drop back on reps and/or sets.

REFERENCES

1. Baley, James. *Illustrated Guide to Developing Strength, Power, and Agility.* Parker Publishing Co. Inc., West Nyack, NY, 1977.
2. Darden, Ellington. *Especially for Women.* Leisure Press, West Point, NY, 1977.
3. Riley, Daniel. *Maximum Muscular Fitness.* Leisure Press, West Point, NY, 1982.
4. Sheffield, Emilyn. *Total Fitness for Women.* Goodyear Publishing Co., Santa Monica, CA, 1980.
5. Tuten, Rich; Moore, Clancy; and Knight, Virgil. *Weight Training Everyone.* Hunter Textbooks Inc., Winston-Salem, NC, 1982.
6. Westcott, Wayne. *Strength Fitness.* Allyn & Bacon, Inc. Boston, 1982.

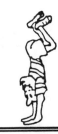

Chapter Eight

CONCERNS FOR SPECIFIC POPULATIONS

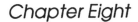

The benefits of exercise are universal and people of all sizes, shapes and ages are reaping the benefits of being physically fit. There are, however, those who need special consideration to get these benefits. Included among these are pregnant women, the elderly, and the young. Each of these populations has specific needs and for them to reach their fitness goals, traditional concepts of exercise may need to be altered.

PREGNANCY

Many women who are regular exercisers want to continue exercising when they become pregnant while others want to begin an exercise program. Exercise during pregnancy can provide many benefits both psychological and physical. According to Pat J. Kulpa, M.D., an expert in the area of exercise and pregnancy, low-risk pregnant women who exercise regularly not only maintain their pre-pregnancy level of fitness, but also obtain a significant training effect (4). Even though most authorities agree that exercise during pregnancy is not harmful, there are still some unanswered questions regarding its effects during pregnancy. Most professionals agree that there is no reason to tell a low-risk, healthy pregnant woman not to exercise but the safety and well-being of the fetus as well as the mother are always a primary concern. Exercise programs for pregnant women should be individualized and the level of fitness should be a major consideration. Exercise during pregnancy helps a woman through the emotional and physical adjustments that have to be made and a well-guided exercise program will improve self-image, relieve muscular tension, and decrease the discomfort of low back pain.

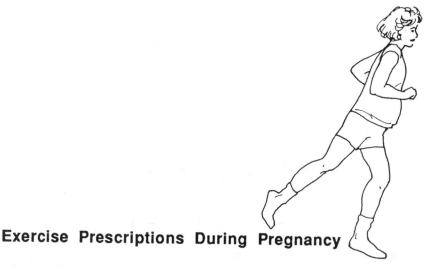

Exercise Prescriptions During Pregnancy

It is important for the pregnant woman to recognize that there will be some limitations imposed by the pregnancy and prudent decisions and basic guidelines should be followed. The exercise prescription should be directed at *maintaining* physical fitness within the limitations of the pregnancy, and because of the variation in heart rate responses it is inappropriate to determine any target zone. Pregnant women are also less efficient in performing physical activities because of their lower cardiac reserve, which is caused by the increase in blood volume, cardiac output and resting heart rate. The following recommendations should be practiced:

1. Avoid exercise during hot or humid days
2. Maintain adequate fluid intake
3. Stop frequently to rest
4. Maintain an adequate diet
5. Rest after activity

Cardiorespiratory activities such as walking, swimming, cycling and low-impact aerobics can be a part of the exercise program. More strenuous activities such as marathon running, hiking, and competitive tennis may cause variation in heart rate and put too much strain on ligaments and joints.

If you have been sedentary, it is strongly recommended that you do not start a strenuous exercise program after becoming pregnant. A low-impact aerobic routine or walking are appropriate ways to begin exercising. If you have been training at high intensity, it is best to gradually reduce the intensity. During vigorous exercise, oxygen is delivered to skeletal muscles for energy and if the uterine blood flow is reduced, the fetus may suffer from oxygen deprivation. Most authorities agree that the heart rate should not exceed 160 beats per minute during high intensity activity.

While exercising, you should drink plenty of fluids to keep the body hydrated and lower the risk of hyperthermia (elevated body temperature). The body temperature of an exercising, pregnant woman should not exceed 101 degrees Fahrenheit. If necessary, exercise should be stopped to replenish fluids.

The following guidelines established by the American College of Obstetricians and Gynecologists and can serve as standards for exercise during pregnancy (14).

1. Regular exercise is recommended over intermittent activity throughout pregnancy and competitive sports should be avoided.

2. Exercise should be performed slowly and carefully because of the shift in the center of gravity. As pregnancy progresses, the center of gravity moves forward causing balance problems. Pregnant women should warmup for longer periods of time to reduce the risk of injury. Jumping jacks and high leg kicks should be avoided.

3. Ballistic type movements or quick change of direction should be eliminated because of connective tissue laxity. Deep flexion and extension of the joints should be avoided because of this laxity. Stretches should not be taken to the point of maximum resistance and when changing positions for various stretches,the pregnant woman should move slowly to make adjustments to the shift in weight.

4. Avoid or eliminate any exercise that might cause abdominal trauma. Exercise should not be done in the supine position (lying down) after the fourth month of pregnancy because in the supine position, the uterus may rest on the aorta and reduce the blood flow to that area. Do not hold your breath during exercise to avoid inducing the Valsalva maneuver which exerts force with the epiglottis closed thereby increasing pressure in the thorax and elevating arterial pressure. When released, the blood pressure drops and dizziness may occur.

5. Calorie intake should be sufficient to accommodate the extra energy needs of pregnancy. Women who exercise need to consume enough calories and nutrients to supply energy for the exercise program and also to provide for a healthy weight gain for the child.

Maintaining physical fitness during pregnancy will enable the pregnant woman to perform everyday activities with less discomfort. Being fit does not imply that a womans labor will be shorter or easier, but there is a dramatic improvement in recuperation time after delivery (14). The return of strength and stamina is much faster and is advantageous in helping the mother cope with the demands of a new baby. However, if at any time during an exercise program, the following conditions occur, stop exercising immediately and consult a physician:
   • Pain or discomfort in any part of the body
   • Menstrual cramping or vaginal bleeding
   • Breathlessness or dizziness
   • Rapid heart rate or irregular heart beat

WARM-UP

All-over Body Stretch
With legs in parallel position, knees should be placed directly over toes. Press forward with the arms. Round the back and shoulders. Relax and repeat.

Calf Stretch

Assume a lunge position. Knee should be placed directly over the feet. Buttocks should be tucked and the hips square. Hold the stretch and repeat other side.

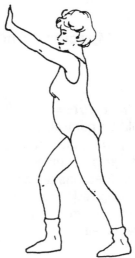

LOW-IMPACT AEROBICS

Caution: One foot should remain on the floor at all times. Minimize jumping.

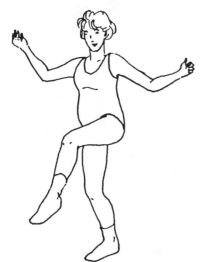

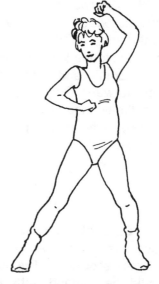

Elbow to Knee Lifts

Knees should be slightly apart. Bring opposite elbow to the knee. Alternate sides and repeat.

Side Lunge with Arm Swings

Feet should be parallel and shoulder-width apart. Lunge to side using upper body movements when appropriate.

Muscular Endurance Exercises

Chest Press

Feet should be parallel, shoulder-width apart. Pelvis should be tucked, arms shoulder distance apart. Press the arms together, creating resistance with the muscles. Return to starting position and repeat.

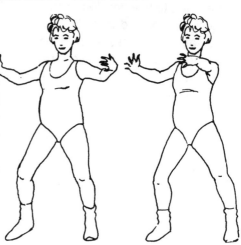

Pelvic Tilt

Place the legs comfortably apart. Inhale and round the back, holding onto the legs for support. Exhale and extend the body forward, pressing the chest through the legs. Return the body to the starting position and repeat.

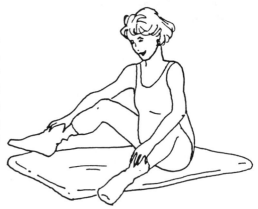

Catback Stretch

Place the arms comfortably under the shoulders. The head should be aligned with the spine. Contract and arch the back, maintaining body alignment. Return to the starting position and repeat the exercise.

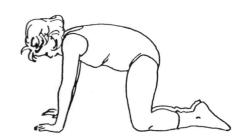

THE ELDERLY

Age should never be viewed as a limiting factor in starting an exercise program. Participation in a regular exercise routine can be very beneficial to people of all ages, and it is especially important for the elderly. Unfortunately, too few older people participate in such programs. This may be attributed to the concern many elderly people have regarding the risk of injury, the chances of experiencing a heart attack, and their doubts about the effect of exercise on their cardiovascular condition and general health.

Exercise Prescription

Although the benefits of exercise are basically the same for the young as they are for the elderly, the prescription for fitness is somewhat different. To experience the aerobic effect, a young healthy adult must exercise three times per week for thirty minutes, at an intensity equal to 70-85 percent of their maximum. For the elderly, the prescription is the same with one major change, the intensity. It is recommended that 40-70 percent be used as the criterion rather than 70-85 percent (13).

Aerobic exercise can retard the aging process by slowing the decline in physical work capacity. This was demonstrated in a recent study comparing the effects of aerobic exercise on men over age 60 and men age 35. It was found that the physical work capacity of the 60 year olds was similar to that of the 35 year olds. Thus, the usual decline in physical work capacity seen with advancing age may be altered by habitual physical activity (13).

Guidelines established for young adults may be useful in designing an aerobics program for the elderly. The major focus should be on keeping the intensity lowered. Anyone over 50 years of age who has been relatively inactive should have a complete physical examination including an exercise stress test. If an individual has been completely sedentary, it is a good idea to start slowly by adding an activity to the daily routine like walking to places where they usually drive. Older people should bend and stretch as often as possible to keep the body limber and responsive to movement.

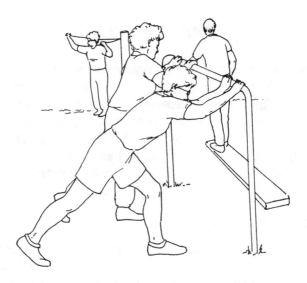

Water activities can be beneficial for the elderly, especially those suffering from arthritis. It should be noted that heart rate levels are lower in the water; in some cases by as much as 20 beats per minute. Thus heart rates should be adjusted downward for water activities. In addition to water activities, women who are predisposed to osteoporosis should include some type of weight-bearing activity to their fitness program.

The elderly have less heat and cold tolerance; therefore, summer exercise programs should be conducted in facilities with good air-conditioning or done outside in the early morning or late evening when it is cooler. Water should be taken as frequently as possible to avoid dehydration in the heat. In cold weather, there is blood vessel constriction and a potential increase in blood pressure; therefore, appropriate clothing and adequate facilities are important considerations. Many elderly persons have become involved in walking programs in shopping malls throughout the country where the air temperature is always comfortably controlled.

When considering the ingredients of a quality aerobics program for the elderly, none is more important than the instructor. An effective exercise leader must be aware of the nature and needs of the elderly and be able to motivate them to exercise. The instructor also has the responsibility to teach them about the values of regular exercise and to remind them that exercise has emotional, psychological and social benefits to compliment the physical benefits.

CHILDREN

There are many benefits to be derived from exercise and the sooner you get started the better. Two of the most important are the reduced chances of coronary heart disease and obesity during adulthood. According to the American Heart Association, it is not uncommon to find coronary risk factors such as elevated cholesterol levels, hypertension, and obesity among children in elementary school. Most health professionals agree that when risk factors appear in childhood, the chances of developing heart disease in adulthood are very good.

How fat you will be as an adult is also determined to a large degree during childhood. According to some experts, fat cells increase in number during the first few years of life and continue through elementary school and conclude with the growth spurt of adolescence. Most non-fat adults have about 25 billion fat cells in their bodies compared with the obese who have approximately three times that many. The fewer fat cells you take into adulthood the better chance you have of avoiding the problems of obesity. Research has made it clear that physically active non-obese children actually consume more calories than their obese inactive counterparts, clearly indicating the need for regular physical activity for children.

Exercise Prescription

Children are not as active as they appear to be and do not voluntarily engage in high intensity aerobic activity (6). Interestingly enough, children and adolescents are the most physiologically fit of any age group (12). Even aerobically untrained children have a capacity for aerobic endurance activities.

Children should be encouraged to exercise at an intensity capable of providing the aerobic effect. This can be done by computing the target heart rate with the necessary adjustment for the higher resting rate of children. Since the resting heart rate of a child is approximately 85, and the theoretical maximum is 205, the application of the target heart rate formula for 60 percent of maximum would be 160 beats per minute.

While children should be encouraged to participate in aerobic activity, there is some concern about the effect of competitive running on the musculoskeletal system. The concern is that the growth center may be damaged and cause stunted growth or uneven development of the knee or hip joints. Therein lies the argument for discouraging children from playing contact sports.

Another consideration for children during aerobic activity is heat intolerance. Children have a less efficient heat dissipation mechanism than adults and, in effect, generate more heat with fewer sweat glands.

Physical education programs should be reinforced at home by family participation in some form of regular activity. This will help children perceive aerobic exercising as an integral part of daily life and cause them to become regular exercising adults.

QUESTIONS AND ANSWERS

Will exercise during pregnancy cause a miscarriage?
There is no basis for this assumption because the fetus is protected by the pelvis and stomach muscles.

If I am a regular exerciser, do I still need to check with the doctor when I become pregnant?
Yes. It is always important to check with the doctor for guidelines regarding exercise during pregnancy.

Are there specific exercises that I should avoid during pregnancy?
Do not perform double leg lifting or any exercise that places stress on the abdominals or lower back.

Is a high-intensity aerobic class appropriate for me if I am considered a low-risk pregnancy?

A low-intensity class might be more appropriate and more comfortable during pregnancy. Dehydration and an increase in body temperature are two important concerns for pregnant women during an aerobic dance class.

Should I diet during pregnancy?

The best outcome for your baby will occur if you gain 20 to 30 pounds during your pregnancy. Eat more if you're exercising. The time to diet is before you become pregnant.

Should I stop exercising during my last month of pregnancy?

If the doctor recommends that you do so because of obstetrical complications.

Will exercise make my labor easier?

Unfortunately, there is no conclusive evidence that indicates this is true. However, being in shape provides extra stamina necessary for delivering a baby.

Can exercise cause me to have a heart attack?

The only way exercise can cause you to have a heart attack is if you have heart disease. A healthy heart can only benefit from a sensible program of aerobic exercise. People who have heart attacks while exercising would experience the same heart attack if their heart rate was elevated by an emotional or non-exercising experience.

Can exercise help delay the aging process?

Exercise cannot prevent the aging process from occurring. However, it can delay some of the effects of aging and research has indicated that older men and women are similar to youth in their ability to improve fitness through exercise.

Is walking the only safe exercise for older adults?

No. It has been shown that with proper guidelines, older adults can participate in all forms of physical activity.

Will an aerobic exercise class improve my body composition even if I am over fifty?

Yes. An aerobic exercise class improves body composition by maintaining lean body mass, increasing the basal metabolic rate, and decreasing body fat.

If I have been diagnosed as having osteoporosis, can I still participate in a traditional, high impact class?

No. If you have been diagnosed as having osteoporosis, you should minimize impact because of the potential it has for aggravating the condition.

Is it dangerous for children to engage in endurance or aerobic type activity?

No. Aerobic exercise is a significant factor in reducing the problems of obesity in adulthood, as well as preventing the risks of coronary heart disease. Furthermore, children who participate in rigorous exercise programs function better physiologically in regular aerobic activity.

Are there any special benefits to be gained by children participating in regular aerobic activity?

Emphatically, yes. Children should be encouraged to run, cycle, swim, walk, and dance. These activities provide physiological and psychological benefits for life.

Should a child eat differently when participating in intense aerobic activity?

Generally speaking, the best way to judge a childs food and fluid intake is to observe the energy level. If performance and energy appear different, it may be necessary to increase the water and food intake.

Are there any negative effects of aerobics for children?

Aerobic exercise is a positive experience which affects children in much the same way as it does adults. Children who engage in regular aerobic exercise programs are less likely to develop coronary artery disease and have problems with obesity in adult life.

REFERENCES

1. Artal , R. "Exercises in Pregnancy," *Sportsmedicine Digest* 9 (5):1, 1987.
2. Bonen, A. and Keizer, H. "Athletic Menstrual Cycle Irregularities: Endocrine Response to Exercise and Training,"*The Physician and Sportsmedicine*12 (8):78, 1984.
3. Brehm, B.A. "How to Give Safe Counsel to Your Pregnant Exercisers," *Fitness Management*. 4 (6):19, 1988.
4. Gauthier, M.M. "Guidelines for Exercises During Pregnancy". *The Physician and Sportsmedicine*. 14 (8):162, 1986.
5. Getchell, B. *Physical Fitness: A Way of Life*. Wiley and Sons, NY, 1983.
6. Gilman, T.B. "Exercise Programs for Children: A Way to Prevent Heart Disease," *The Physician and Sportsmedicine* 12 (9):96, 1982.
7. Greenburg, J.S. and Pargman, D. *Physical Fitness: A Wellness Approach.* Prentice Hall, Englewood Cliffs, NJ,1986.
8. Hage, P. "Diet and Exercise Programs for Coronary Heart Disease: Better Late Than Never," *The Physician and Sportsmedicine* 10 (9):121, 1982.
9. Hobson, A.J. and Robinson, J.P. *Aerobic Dance for Effective Performance.* Kendall Hunt Pub. Co. Dubuque, IA, 1987.
10. Miller, D.K. and Allen, T.E. *Fitness: A Lifetime Commitment.* Burgess Publishing Co., Minneapolis, 1986.
11. Piscopo, J. *Fitness and Aging.* Wiley and Sons. New York,1985.
12. Rowland, T.W. and Hoontis, P.P. "Organizing Road Races for Children: Special Concerns." *The Physician and Sportsmedicine* 13 (3):126, 1985.
13. Sager, K. "Senior Fitness for the Health of It,"*The Physician and Sportsmedicine.*11 (10):31, 1983.
14. Wallace, J. "Exercise and Pregnancy: Physiological Considerations," *International Dance-Exercise Association Instructor's Manual.* Idea Publications. San Diego,1987.

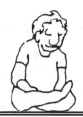

Chapter Nine

Food for Thought
THE ROLE OF NUTRITION

If you are truly serious about achieving a high level of personal fitness, then it is imperative that you not only understand the role of nutrition but apply the principles of proper nutrition to your daily eating plan. To train hard to improve your fitness but neglect the rules of good nutrition is to automatically limit the potential for improvement. You can only hope to achieve your optimal level of fitness through a combined program of well-planned exercise and attention to the fundamentals of good nutrition. Actually, proper nutrition forms the foundation of physical performance. It provides the fuel for work and the elements for utilizing the potential energy contained within this fuel. Perhaps the importance of under-standing nutrition is best stated by Dr. Jean Mayer, one of the country's most respected authorities on nutrition: "Most of the major causes of death and disability — heart disease and stroke, high blood pressure, adult onset diabetes, liver and kidney diseases — either result from faulty nutrition or from a combination of factors that include poor nutrition. . . A few simple changes in the American diet and habits of life could greatly reduce the number of people who acquire these diseases and who may die from them."

One of the problems which prevents changes in eating habits is the number of myths, distortions and fallacies surrounding the area of nutrition.

It is difficult for the average individual who does not have the time or resources to determine the actual facts about nutrition. Some of the confusion is caused by hucksters who make claims based on poorly-designed studies which should not be used as a basis for decisions about diet and nutrition. Additional confusion occurs because outdated

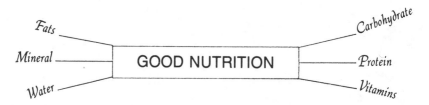

Fats

Mineral

Water

GOOD NUTRITION

Carbohydrate

Protein

Vitamins

information, which has been reversed by more current evidence, is still being used as a basis for decisions. However, the greatest deterrents in sorting myth from fact are the advertising experts who try to influence the uninformed. They use every means possible to confuse the public by quoting studies their researchers have conducted or by belittling the research of the unbiased nutritionists. These large companies would have you believe that not only is nothing harmful in any of their products but that none of the research is conclusive. The end result is that the average individual does not know what to believe and ultimately does nothing to change his/her diet from the typical American diet. This diet is one of the reasons that Americans have such a high rate of heart disease. There is no supplement available which supplies all the nutrients essential to life in the amounts in which they are needed. Also, no single class of foods provides what the body needs to function at a high level.

The goal of this chapter is to help you gain an understanding of nutrition which will enable you to make confident changes in your current eating habits.

UNDERSTANDING THE NUTRIENTS

Nutrients are chemical substances obtained from food during digestion. The body requires six basic nutrients: carbohydrates, proteins, fats, vitamins, minerals and water. It is possible to obtain these nutrients from the foods we eat, however, because of present eating habits, many people lack an adequate supply of one or more of these nutrients. Thus, the first step in analyzing the quality of a diet is to gain a meaningful understanding of the role each nutrient plays in helping us achieve optimal health.

Carbohydrates

There are two categories of carbohydrates—sugars and starches. The confusion and concern about carbohydrates in our diet has developed because of the great variability between these two groups. One group is made up of the sugars that are quickly broken down and absorbed by the body. These simple carbohydrates include refined sugars such as those found in white bread, rolls, snack food, candy bars, jellies, and hot fudge sundaes. In addition, a simple carbohydrate found naturally in fruits is more slowly digested and is packed with vitamins, minerals and fiber.

Complex carbohydrates are those identified as the starches which provide a stable form of energy and also contain other nutrients needed by the body. Complex carbohydrates are generally found in natural foods like vegetables, cereals, whole grains and beans.

Sugar

It is important to realize the potential problems related to refined carbohydrates. In addition to increased dental problems, dietary sugar causes elevation of blood sugar and blood triglycerides, and may stimulate the liver to produce more cholesterol. Because sugar is quickly converted to glucose and is rapidly absorbed into the bloodstream, there may be a short feeling of quick energy. However, the pancreas releases insulin necessary for the utilization of the sugar in such large amounts that the blood sugar level is then driven lower than normal. As a result, you may experience the uncomfortable feeling of hypoglycemia: light-headedness, weakness, depression, and even dizziness.

This condition can be even more serious if large amounts of sugar are ingested throughout a lifetime. This places the cells of the pancreas under constant and abnormal stress which leads either to the exhaustion

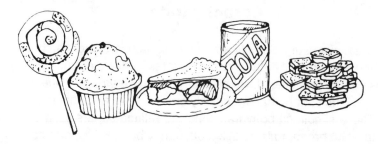

of their ability to synthesize insulin or to the loss of the capacity of tissue cells to absorb the hormone from the bloodstream. In either case, the end result can be adult onset diabetes.

Part of the problem with the high intake of refined sugar is the "hidden" sugar in so many foods. Processed foods and beverages account for more than two-thirds of the refined sugar consumed. One might be surprised to read the label of many foods and find that sugar has been added. There is also confusion as to whether honey, brown sugar, and molasses are better substitutes for table sugar. For all purposes, honey is still straight sugar, brown sugar is just white sugar with molasses, and raw sugar is no longer available on the market. Blackstrap molasses is the only sugar with anything to offer of nutritional value. It does contain some minerals from the original sugar cane, plus calcium and iron from the processing.

Most people would be wise to observe the following methods of decreasing sugar intake:

1. Drink fewer soft drinks (they average 8 teaspoons per 12 ounces).
2. Eat fewer baked goods and, when cooking your own, decrease the sugar content.
3. Read labels and avoid foods containing added sugar.

Fiber

Another important component of complex carbohydrates is fiber or roughage. Fiber is the structural part of plants which is neither digested nor absorbed by the body. Dietary fiber is what is left over when food is digested in the human digestive tract. Fiber's most important role is to serve as an intestinal "housecleaner." The added bulk supplied by fiber makes the intestines contract which speeds the food through the digestive system. Since toxic chemicals, including some carcinogens (cancer-causing), can be produced by bacteria and enzymes during digestion, this shorter "transit time" helps to move them out faster, perhaps averting cancer of the colon. High-fiber diets also cause the cholesterol to bind with bile acids and then be excreted, which causes a decrease in blood cholesterol level.

Foods that are especially good sources of fiber include bran, oats, wheat, corn, apples, cabbage, potatoes, turnips, raspberries, black-berries, and seeds.

Carbohydrates (Complex)

Function	Style	Calories Per Gram	%Recommended In Diet
Broken down into glucose, which is the major source of energy. Some is stored in liver and muscles in the form of glycogen. Supply fiber.	Fruits Vegetables Grains Cereals	4	58% or higher

Note: Limit your intake of refined carbohydrates such as table sugar, sweets, pastries, and soft drinks.

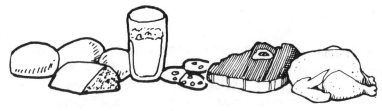

Proteins

Proteins are made up of amino acids needed to build, repair and regulate the function of the body's cells. The body can manufacture some amino acids but not all. Those which must be supplied by the foods we eat each day are known as essential amino acids. Protein foods that contain all the essential amino acids are called complete proteins and are generally foods of animal origin. Those protein foods lacking in certain essential amino acids are referred to as incomplete proteins. However, two or more incomplete proteins can be combined to form a complete protein.

The key factor is providing the body with a variety of foods in a relatively balanced diet. If this occurs, the body has the ability to accommodate wide variations in the type and amount of protein it receives and still meet its needs. As a rule, Americans actually consume too much protein. Only 10-12% of the total calories eaten per day should be from protein.

Proteins

Function	Source	Calories Per Gram	%Recom- mended In Diet
Important for growth maintenance and repair of tissue. Also used to form hormones and enzymes; additional source of energy	*Complete Proteins:* cheese, eggs, milk chicken, fish, meat. *Incomplete Proteins:* dried peas, beans legumes, black-eyed peas, soybeans, black beans.	4	10-12%

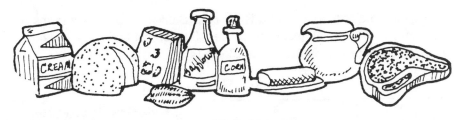

Fats

Some fats are needed by the body because they fulfill several important functions. However, the typical American diet contains over 40% fat as compared to the 20-30% which is currently recommended. In addition, it is important to examine the types of fat included in your diet.

The basic building blocks are fatty acids. The fatty acids combine with glycerol to form glycerides. When glycerol combines with three fatty acids, it forms triglycerides. The classification of fats is also based on the number of hydrogen atoms combined with the carbon atoms. Saturated fats have the maximum number of hydrogen atoms, and they remain hard at room temperature. Hydrogenation is a process in which a fat or oil is made to react with hydrogen. This results in a more stable fat and is used to convert a liquid polyunsaturated oil to a more solid form. It does not necessarily increase its saturation.

Those fatty acids which the human body requires but cannot produce are called essential fatty acids. They are polyunsaturated fats and can be obtained primarily from vegetable oils. Linoleic acid, the most important essential fatty acid, should provide about 2% of the calories in the diet.

Actually, all fats are a mixture of saturated, polyunsaturated and mono-unsaturated fatty acids. But some foods are higher in one than the other and it is important to know these differences. Dietary rules recommend that only 10% of the calories in your diet come from saturated fats. So much "invisible" fat is in foods that many people are unaware of just how much they are getting. This is now recognized as a major health problem because every population in the world having a high rate of heart disease eats a diet rich in saturated fat and cholesterol. It has been found that saturated fat is the prime influence on blood cholesterol level — one gram raises it twice as much as an equal amount of polyunsaturated fat.

Another major health hazard is cancer. Studies now link six forms of cancer with dietary fat, including cancer of the breast and colon — two of the top cancer killers in the United States (4).

Fats

Function	Source	Calories Per Gram	%Recommended in Diet
Part of the structure of every cell Stored energy Supplies essential fatty acids Provides and carries fat-soluble vitamins A, D, E, K	*Unsaturated:*Safflower oil, Corn oil,Sunflower oil, Soybean oil,Margarines (made with vegetable oils). *Saturated:* Solid and hydrogenated shortening,Coconut oil,Cocoa butter,Palm oil,Butter,Cheese,Meat,Milk. *Monounsaturated:* Olive oil,Peanut oil.	9	20-30% 10% polyunsaturated 10% monounsaturared

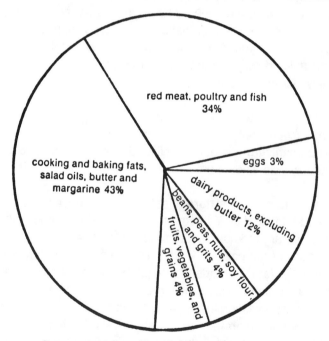

red meat. poultry and fish 34%

cooking and baking fats, salad oils, butter and margarine 43%

eggs 3%

dairy products, excluding butter 12%

beans, peas, nuts, soy flour, and grits 4%

fruits, vegetables, and grains 4%

Sources of Fat in the American Diet

''Nutrient Content of the National Food Supply,'' R. Marston, L. Page. *National Food Review,* pp. 28-33, U.S. Department of Agriculture, December 1978.

Cholesterol

Cholesterol is a waxy, fatty-like material utilized by the body in many chemical processes. Even though cholesterol has no calories as fat does, scientists often refer to it as a fat because it has similar effects on the body. Cholesterol has many important functions in the body: it is a key part of brain tissue, it helps protect nerve fibers, it is necessary for sex hormones as well as other hormones, it helps make Vitamin D, and it is necessary for the membranes of all body cells. Actually, cholesterol is such a vital substance that almost every cell in the body manufactures it.

Cholesterol is carried through the blood by a series of molecules called lipoproteins. The low density lipoproteins (LDLs) pick up cholesterol that originates from our diet or is manufactured in the liver and deposits it in the cells for processing. If there is more cholesterol than is needed for daily metabolism, the LDLs may deposit this fatty cargo on the lining of the arteries. These deposits can narrow the arteries in the heart and cause a fatty plaque build-up. This not only causes the heart to strain, but may cause a clot to dislodge and flow through the bloodstream. This clot may eventually lodge in a coronary artery causing reduction of blood flow to the heart muscle and perhaps death from a heart attack. However, high density lipoproteins float around in the bloodstream and pick up the excess cholesterol and carry it back to the liver for excretion from the body. Obviously, our goal is to try to increase our levels of HDL in the blood which can be done by:
1. Eating a low fat, low cholesterol diet
2. Engaging in aerobic exercise
3. Not smoking
4. Avoiding obesity

It is important to point out that the effects of cholesterol consumption vary from person to person. Some individuals may be lucky enough to maintain a low blood cholesterol level regardless of their diet, but these people are definitely the exception to the rule. Obviously there are many factors that can influence one's blood cholesterol level, and we presently do not completely understand how a change in this level can be brought about. It does not seem, for instance, that a high dietary intake will depress the body's synthesis of cholesterol to the point that it will cancel out the effect of diet. Some studies now reveal that stress causes an increase in cholesterol production and that a Vitamin C deficiency inhibits the removal of cholesterol from the blood as it passes through the liver.

In regard to an optimal level for blood cholesterol, it seems that below 180 (per 100ml of blood) your risk of heart disease is low. This risk starts to rise slowly with increasing blood cholesterol levels. Above a level of 250, your heart attack risk jumps sharply. However, no blood cholesterol level is guaranteed to prevent a heart attack. It is not now possible to draw a line between safe and unsafe. We can predict that the chances or odds of suffering a heart attack rise as the cholesterol level rises (4).

Another important consideration is the ratio between your total cholesterol and the HDL cholesterol. Most authorities recommend that men keep the ratio of total cholesterol to HDL cholesterol below 4.6 and women keep the ratio below 4.0.

Although we still have many unanswered questions, most research has shown that a low-fat, low cholesterol diet may be the best way to prevent heart disease. The following agencies have determined that there is enough evidence to strongly advocate this diet for all Americans: U.S. Dept. of Agriculture, Dept. of Health, Education, and Welfare, Senate Select Committee on Nutrition & Human Needs, American Heart Association, American Health Association, National Heart, Lung and Blood Institute, and Center for Science in the Public Interest.

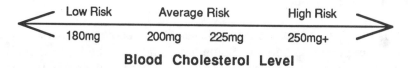

Blood Cholesterol Level

The only foods high in cholesterol are those from animal sources. Therefore, a low cholesterol intake involves **lowering** your consumption of the following: eggs (no more than 3 per week), shrimp, caviar, red meat, all organ and gland meats. In addition, saturated fats such as coconut oil, butterfat, and palm oil raise cholesterol levels.

The chart which follows, shows the typical sources of cholesterol in our diet and the specific count found in a number of common foods.

CHOLESTEROL LEVELS

Mg.	Food	Mg.	Food	Mg.	Food
35	Butter, 1 T	22	Butter, whipped, 1 T	24	Blue Cheese, 1 oz.
28	Cheddar cheese, 1 oz.	23	Low-fat cottage	48	Creamed cottage
13	Uncreamed cottage		cheese, 1 cup		cheese, 1 cup
	cheese, 1 cup	16	Cream cheese, 1 T	27	Mozzarella, 1 oz.
18	Mozzarella, part-skim, 1 oz.	35	Swiss cheese, 1-1/4 oz.	8	Sour Cream, 1 T
252	Egg, whole	53	Ice cream, 1 cup	26	Ice Milk, 1 cup
34	Milk, 1 cup	22	Milk, low-fat (2%), 1 cup	5	Milk, non-fat, 1 cup
3	Skim milk, 1 cup	80	Beef, 3 oz.	63	Chicken, 1/3 breast
114	Clams, 1 cup	34	Frankfurter, 2	83	Lamb, 3 oz.
372	Liver, 3 oz.	123	Lobster, 1 cup	120	Oysters, 1 cup
90	Pork, 3 oz.	192	Shrimp, 1 cup	102	Tuna, 1 can
65	Turkey, light, 3 oz.	86	Turkey, dark, 3 oz.	0	Margarine
79	Milk, evaporated, 1 cup	105	Milk, condensed, 1 cup	10	Mayonnaise, 1 T
17	Yogurt, non-fat, 8 oz.				

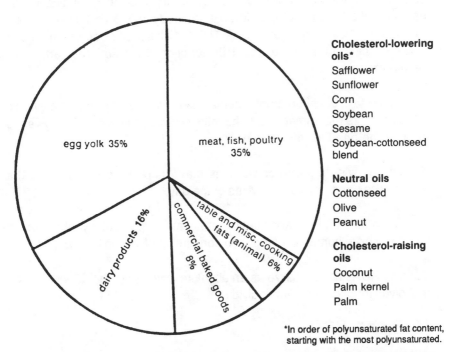

Cholesterol-lowering oils*

Safflower
Sunflower
Corn
Soybean
Sesame
Soybean-cottonseed blend

Neutral oils

Cottonseed
Olive
Peanut

Cholesterol-raising oils

Coconut
Palm kernel
Palm

*In order of polyunsaturated fat content, starting with the most polyunsaturated.

SOURCES OF CHOLESTEROL IN THE AMERICAN DIET
Based on Stamler, J., in *Reprints from Ischaemic Heart Disease*, FADL-Forlag, 1977

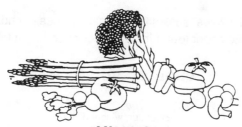

Vitamins

A vitamin is an organic substance essential for the body to perform its complex chemical reactions. Vitamins cannot be synthesized by the body and are not nutrients in the sense of supplying energy or building tissue, but they aid in the utilization and absorption of the nutrients. Each vitamin performs one or more specific functions in the body. Vitamins are divided into two groups on the basis of their solubility. The fat-soluble vitamins A, D, E, and K, are those found in foods associated with fats. They tend to remain stored in the body in moderate quantities. The water soluble vitamins are B and C and are transported in the fluids of the tissues and cells and are not stored in the body in appreciable quantities. The chart which follows on pages 140-141 describes each vitamin and gives specific information about its function, best sources, and daily requirements.

An important question many people ask is whether the use of a vitamin supplement is recommended. The following reasons have been given to support the need for a supplement:

1. The body's demand for vitamins may increase depending on the stresses and physical activities of the day.

2. One's intake of dietary vitamins may vary — particularly when eating away from home, smoking, and consuming alcoholic beverages.

3. The RDAs cannot serve as an absolute indicator of the adequacy of a given intake for a given individual.

MDR and RDA

As a guide to an adequate intake of the various nutrients, the Minimum Daily Requirement (MDR) and Recommended Dietary Allowance (RDA) have been established. The MDRs were established by the Food and Drug Administration and are average levels, with a small safety margin, required to prevent symptoms of actual deficiency. The RDAs were developed by the Food and Nutrition Board of the National Academy of Sciences and are higher than the MDRs. Actually a reliable test for determining individual requirements has not yet been devised.

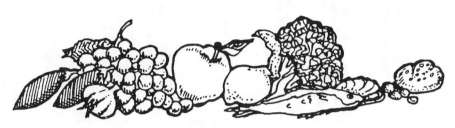

Minerals

Minerals are inorganic nutrients which are important in activating numerous reactions that release energy during the breakdown of carbohydrates, proteins, and fats. There are six macrominerals required in larger quantities than the others: sodium, potassium, chloride, calcium, phosphorus, and magnesium. These are needed in the diet in amounts of 100 mg. or more per day. There are 14 others, called trace minerals, which are required in amounts from 100 mg. per day to a few micrograms.

Minerals are supplied by the foods we eat and by the water we drink. The quantities needed are small: the total amount of minerals needed in a day is approximately 200 mg., which could be the size of a pea or a small pill, while those needed in the microgram range could be as tiny as a grain of sand.

The following chart describes each mineral and provides information about its function, sources, and RDA.

VITAMIN INFORMATION

Vitamin	Food Sources	Deficiency Effect	Function	RDA (Adults)
A	Fish-liver oils, liver, butter, cream, whole milk, whole-milk cheeses, egg yolk, dark-green leafy vegetables, yellow fruits and vegetables.	Night blindness, eye inflammation, dry, rough skin, reduced resistance to infection.	Needed for normal vision. Protects against night blindness. Keeps skin and mucous membranes resistant to infection.	5000 IU
B Complex B₁ (Thiamine)	Pork, liver, organ meats, brewer's yeast, wheat germ, whole-grain cereals and breads, enriched cereals and breads, soybeans, peanuts and other legumes, milk.	Beriberi.	Promotes normal appetite and digestion. Necessary for a healthy nervous system.	1.5 mg.
B₂ (Riboflavin)	Milk, powdered whey, liver, organ meats, meats, eggs, leafy green vegetables, dried yeast, enriched foods.	Cracks at corners of mouth, inflamed, sore lips, inflamed, discolored tongue, dermatitis, anemia.	Helps cells use oxygen. Helps maintain good vision. Needed for good skin.	1.7 mg.
Niacin	Lean meat, fish, poultry, liver, kidney, whole-grain and enriched cereals and breads, green vegetables, peanuts, brewer's yeast.	Pellagra.	Aids metabolism of proteins, carbos, fats.	20 mg.
Pantothenic Acid	Present in most plant and animal tissue, liver, kidney, yeast, eggs, peanuts, whole-grain cereals, beef, tomatoes, broccoli, salmon.	(Rare) Gastrointestinal disturbance, depression, confusion.	Necessary for metabolism of proteins, carbos, fats.	10 mg.
B₆ (Pyridoxine)	Wheat germ, meat, liver, kidney, whole-grain cereals, soybeans, peanuts, corn.	(Rare) Inflamed mouth and tongue, depression, irritability, convulsions.	Maintains normal hemoglobin (carries oxygen to tissues).	2.0 mg.
Biotin	Liver, sweetbreads, yeast, eggs, legumes.	(Extremely rare) Inflamed skin, hair loss, lethargy, loss of appetite.	Coenzyme, functions in metabolism of major nutrients.	0.3 mg.

VITAMIN INFORMATION, cont'd

Vitamin	Food Sources	Deficiency Effect	Function	RDA (Adult)
Folic Acid	Widespread in liver, kidney, yeast, deep-green leafy vegetables.	Anemia, stunted growth, damage to lining of small intestine.	Maintains normal hemoglobin.	.04 mg.
B₁₂ (Cyanocobalamin)	Animal protein.	Pernicious anemia, stunted growth.	Maintains normal hemoglobin.	6 mcg.
C (Ascorbic Acid)	Citrus fruits, tomatoes, strawberries, cantaloupe, cabbage, broccoli, kale, potatoes.	Scurvy.	Maintains cementing material that holds the body cells together. Needed for healthy gums. Helps body resist infection.	60 mg.
D	Fish-liver oils, fortified milk, activated sterols, exposure to sunlight.	Rickets, osteomalacia (loss of calcium from bones in adults).	Builds strong bones and teeth. Aids calcium absorption.	400 IU
E (Tocopherol)	Plant tissues, wheat germ oil, vegetable oils, nuts, legumes.	Unknown in persons eating normal, mixed diet.	Not fully understood. Works as anti-oxidant.	15 IU
K	Green leaves such as spinach, cabbage, cauliflower.	Excessive bleeding.	Aids blood-clotting.	300-500 mcg.

Adapted from the following sources: 1980 Recommended Daily Dietary Allowances, Food and Nutrition Board, National Academy of Sciences — National Research Council; *Runner's World*, April 1981.

MINERAL REQUIREMENTS

MINERALS	WHAT IT DOES	R.D.A.	GOOD SOURCES	
CALCIUM	Developing & maintaining strong bones & teeth — normal blood clotting, heartbeat, transmission of nerve impulses, & muscle contraction	800 mg.	milk & milk products green leafy vegetables, almonds	**MACROMINERALS**
PHOSPHORUS	Utilization of energy, muscle action, & nerve transmission. With calcium, essential for formation of bones, & teeth	800 mg.	meat, poultry, fish, eggs, & whole grain foods	
MAGNESIUM	Essential for energy conversions in the body. Helps control muscle contractions.	300 - 350 mg.	dark bread, nuts, green leafy vegetables, dairy products.	
POTASSIUM	With sodium it helps regulate the balance and volume of body fluids.	1875 - 5625 mg.	all fruits & vegetables, pecans & walnuts, wheat germ, soybeans, & molasses	
SODIUM	Found in blood plasma & other fluids outside cells — helps to maintain normal water balance	1100 - 3300 mg.	meat, fish, poultry, eggs, and milk	
CHLORIDE (Mainly in compound form with sodium or potassium)	Regulates correct balance of acid & alkali in blood. Stimulates production of hydrochloric acid in stomach for disgestion	1700 - 5100 mg.	table salt, kelp, ripe olives & rye flour	
IRON	Red Blood Cell Formation	18 mg.	eggs, liver, whole grains, dried fruits & legumes	**TRACE**
ZINC	Protein synthesis, growth, and development	15 mg.	fish, beef, chicken, whole grains, vegetables, & oysters	
IODINE	Functioning of thyroid gland (breathing rate of tissues)	150 mcg.	seafoods	
COPPER	Action of enzyme systems & normal functioning of central nervous system — Involved with storage & release of iron to form hemoglobin.	2.0 - 3.0 mg.	organ meats, shellfish nuts, & dried legumes	
SELENIUM	Functioning of kidneys, pancreas, and liver.	.05 - 0.2 mg.	organ meats, muscle and seafoods	
MANGANESE	Normal tendon & bone structure	2.5 - 5.0 mg.	peas, beans, nuts, fruits, & whole grains	

Salt

Salt is an essential mineral nutrient composed of sodium and chloride. We need the electrolyte, sodium, to help maintain a proper fluid balance in our blood and tissues and the acid base balance outside the body cells. However, an excessive intake forces the kidneys to work overtime and contributes to bloating, tissue swelling, and menstrual discomforts. In addition, the relationship of salt to the development of high blood pressure is now well documented. Studies show a worldwide correlation between the quantity of salt ingested and the incidence of hypertension in the population. In those countries where a low amount of salt is consumed, there is a corresponding low incidence of hypertension (6). While our actual physiological requirement for sodium is only 220 mg. (or about 1/10 of a teaspoon), the average American consumes 10-20 grams (the equivalent of 2-4 teaspoons) of salt per day.

The problem is that we really can't tell how much salt is in the processed foods we eat. However, we do know that salt is needlessly added to many foods by the processors. This is why canned and ready-to-eat foods increase our sodium intake enormously. Therefore, in order to reduce salt intake we suggest:

1. Reduce use of salt in cooking and at the table.
2. Choose foods that have not been processed (fresh fruits and vegetables).
3. Reduce consumption of foods containing visible salt (potato chips, pretzels, salted nuts, corn chips, etc).
4. Reduce consumption of processed foods such as canned vegetables, snack foods, and frozen dinners (5).

Water

Although water carries no food value, it is essential for transporting materials and provides a medium within the cell in which the cell's chemical reaction takes place. It is recommended that two to three quarts of water be ingested each day to assist in the digestion of food, excretion, glandular secretion, and formation of blood plasma. Water also helps regulate body temperature (by evaporation through the skin).

It is especially important that persons involved in strenuous exercise programs take care to replace the water lost through perspiration. A good rule to follow would be to drink *at least* one large glass of water before and after exercise. Another suggestion is to make it a habit to stop and drink at every water fountain you pass. Of course, under certain circumstances, this could pose a problem.

THE REVISED BASIC FOUR

Nutritionists have now recognized four basic food groups as being the key to obtaining a well-balanced, nutritious diet. Essentially these food groups can still be used as a guideline for proper eating. However, in view of the information now available concerning the possible dangers of some foods, we need to select carefully those that are low in fat, saturated fat, and cholesterol. Although the groups are not new, our emphasis on which foods are given priority has changed. Instead of selecting any of the foods within a group, we suggest that you give careful consideration to your selection. A fifth group has been added because guidelines are needed for certain common foods usually included in most diets.

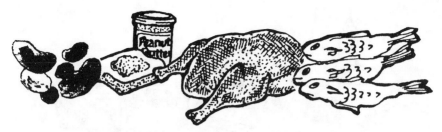

I.   Meat, Poultry, Fish, Eggs, Legumes, Nuts

Eat more poultry. The fat of chicken, turkey, and other fowl is more polyunsaturated than the fat of red meats. Chicken and turkey are very lean if the skin is removed, since much of the fat occurs in the skin.

Eat more fish. No fish has a high saturated fat content.

Eat more beans, peas, and lentils. These provide generous amounts of B vitamins and proteins and have almost no fat and no cholesterol (except soybeans).

Eat nuts, seeds, and peanut butter in moderation. Although the fat content is relatively high, the fat of most nuts and seeds is unsaturated.

Eat fewer egg yolks — limit yourself to two or three per week. Replace fatty meat with lean red meat.

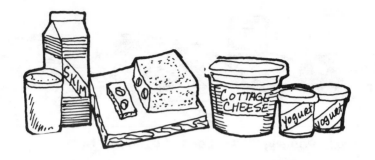

II. Dairy Products: Milk, Cheese, Ice Cream

Use low-fat or skim milk in cooking and drinking.

Use low-fat cottage cheese.

Use less hard cheese. Use part skim cheeses such as Jarlsberg or Mozzarella.

Try making your own low-fat cream cheese, sour cream, and whipped topping with low-fat ingredients.

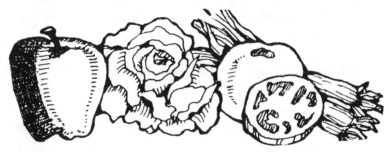

III. Fruits and Vegetables

All fruits and vegetables are cholesterol-free. Most do not have any fat to speak of unless it is added while cooking. Coconut is an exception. It is high in saturated fat. Avocadoes are also high in fat content but it is mostly monounsaturated.

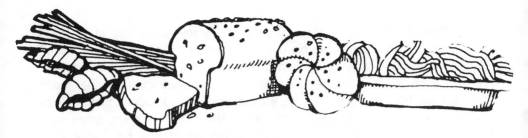

IV. Bread, Grains, and Cereals

Use grains and cereals made from whole wheat flour or lightly milled.

Use any low-fat flour product.

Use pita breads.

Use breads, cereals, crackers, pasta, tortillas, baked goods and other grain products without added fats, oils, sugars, or egg yolks.

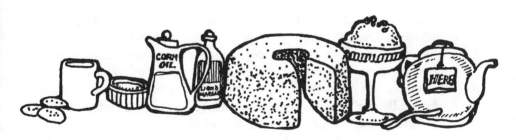

V. The Extras — Fats, Oils, Desserts, and Beverages

Use oils that are highest in polyunsaturated fat: safflower, sunflower, corn oil, etc.

Use diet margarines (half as much fat per tablespoon as regular) and "whipped" margarines.

Avoid all commercial baked goods — make your own low-fat product.

Use cakes and cookies that are low in fat: angel food cake (no fat, no cholesterol), fig bars, and ginger snaps.

Use vegetable juices, unsweetened fruit juices, and herbal tea.

147

One final note on the basic food groups. Many people look at the list of foods we are suggesting be eaten less and remark that all the "good" foods are bad for you. No doubt this does appear to be the case, but once you adjust to these new eating habits you will find that other foods will now become "good" — you will acquire a taste for foods that are **less sweet**, **less salty**, and **less fat**. Also, keep in mind there is a difference in "cutting back" and "cutting out" foods from your diet. Hopefully, once you are able to distinguish the difference between low quality and high quality food, you will make the choice essential for good health.

RECOMMENDED DIETARY GOALS

In 1977 the U.S. Senate Select Committee on Human Nutrition and Human Needs, chaired by Senator George McGovern, issued a statement on risk factors in the American diet and a proposal for changes in eating habits of Americans. This committee recognized that the changes which had been taking place in the American diet for the past fifty years had not been beneficial to the health of the nation. Never before had a government agency made such specific recommendations on what should be eaten. Although these goals were met with considerable resistance when they were first released (by food industries directly affected by the report—meat, eggs, sugar, etc.), they were soon reinforced by similar dietary guidelines issued by the U.S. Department of Agriculture—Health, Education, and Welfare in 1980.

Briefly the "Dietary Goals" for the United States are as follows:
1. Increase consumption of fruits, vegetables, and whole grains.
2. Increase consumption of poultry and fish and decrease consumption of meat.
3. Decrease consumption of foods high in fat, and partially substitute polyunsaturated fat for saturated fat.
4. Substitute nonfat milk for whole milk.
5. Decrease consumption of butter, fat, eggs, and other high cholesterol sources.
6. Decrease consumption of sugar and foods high in sugar content.
7. Decrease consumption of salt and foods high in salt content (2).

THE LAST WORD

We each control the types and amounts of food we eat. Therefore, we are directly responsible for our body's nutritional state. Through better nutrition we can improve the quality of all aspects of our lives. Whether at work, in school, in sports or in leisure activities, we will perform only as well as our physical well-being allows. One cannot consistently deprive the body of the essential nutrients it needs, for the effects of a diet deficiency or imbalance are slow and subtle, but inevitable. The choice of a good diet and improved nutrition is yours.

FOOD SELECTION CHART

ARE YOU MAKING THE BEST CHOICES?

Food Group	Optimal	Adequate	Questionable	Inadequate
Fruits and Vegetables Vitamin A or C Pectic (fiber)	Most fruits and vegetables	Fruit and vegetable juices, dried fruits	Avocados (high fat content)	Vegetables in cream or butter sauce, fried vegetables, olives
Bread and Cereals B Vitamins, Cellulose (fiber), minerals	Whole grains: Shredded wheat, Grape nuts, Nutri-grain, Total, oatmeal, Wheaties; corn, barley, wild rice, brown rice	White rice, white bread, spaghetti, noodles, macaroni, tortillas	cakes, cookies, pies, donuts	sugar, honey
Meat, Poultry, Fish Protein, iron, niacin	Water-packed tuna, beans, legumes, cod, flounder, scallops	chicken- turkey white meat; crab, lobster, oysters, catfish	beef, eggs, ham, liver, lamb, chicken or turkey dark meat, mackerel	bacon, pork, spareribs, sausage, hot dogs, nuts, bologna, pepperoni
Milk and Dairy Products Vitamin B - riboflavin, Protein, Calcium	skim milk, non-fat yogurt, uncreamed cottage cheese, low-fat yogurt	low-fat milk, part-skim mozzarella, creamed cottage cheese	most cheese, whole milk, part-skim ricotta cheese	ice cream, butter, ricotta cheese, eggnog, margarine, mayonnaise

QUESTIONS AND ANSWERS

Why are "fast foods" not recommended?

There are three primary problems associated with eating too much "fast foods": salt, fat, and calories. These foods also contain too much sugar and too little fiber and vitamins.

Are there any dangers in a vegetarian diet?

If one is a strict vegetarian and avoids all milk products as well as meat, there are potential problems. Unless care is taken, protein intake may be insufficient, a calcium deficiency may result, and vitamin B_{12} intake may be inadequate. On the other side of the picture, vegetarians generally have a diet lower in calories and higher in complex carbohydrates and fiber.

Will drinking alcoholic beverages affect my exercise and fitness?

In addition to the serious health hazards associated with alcohol consumption (liver and kidney problems), the following effects on exercise and fitness have been identified:

1. Reduction in the body's ability to utilize oxygen for at least 48 hours after consumption.
2. Intake of empty calories—7 calories per gram with no vitamins and minerals.
3. Potential increase in weight due to the additional calories in the diet.

SUGGESTED LABS

Lab 8 Nutrition and Diet Analysis

REFERENCES

1. Allsen, P., Harrison, J., and Vance, B. *Fitness for Life*. Wm. C. Brown Co., Dubuque, Iowa, 1984.
2. Falls, H., Baylor, A., and Dishman, R. *Essentials of Fitness.* Saunders, Philadelphia, 1980.
3. Garrison, Linda and Reed, Ann. *Fitness for Every Body.* Mayfield Publishing Co., Palo Alto, California, 1980.
4. Hausman, Patricia. *Jack Sprat's Legacy.* Richard Marek Publishing Co., New York, 1981.
5. Kapitan, Anne and Wintle, Carol. *Food for the Health of It.* Somerville Public Schools, Somerville, Massachusetts, 1980.
6. Miller, David K. and Allen, T. Earl. *Fitness: A Lifetime Commitment.* Burgess Publishing Co., Minneapolis, 1986.

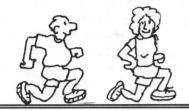

Chapter Ten

The Balancing Act
WEIGHT CONTROL

Knowledge of the basics of nutrition is the first step in learning to eat properly, to attaining (or maintaining) your optimal weight, and to achieving a healthy lifestyle. However, the matter of permanent weight control is not a simple one. This chapter is designed to help you understand the how and why of weight control, and to provide a plan for establishing a program based on your individual needs.

Analyzing Your Body Composition

When it comes to evaluating body composition, scales and height /weight charts can be misleading. All they really say is whether you have excess weight—body weight that exceeds the normal standards based on height, sex, and frame size. They are not adequate because it is not a person's weight, but what that weight consists of that is important—in other words, how much of your weight its lean mass (bone, muscle, water) and how much is fat. A person could be in the acceptable range according to the height/weight tables but have excessive fat, while a muscular person might be considered overweight yet have very little body fat. For a typical height/weight chart which can be used to determine your correct weight, see page 17.

Our major concern should be that of obesity — excess accumulation of body fat beyond what is considered desirable for a person's sex. The amount of fat can be evaluated by measuring certain body areas using an instrument called "calipers" or by doing a simple "pinch" test. These methods are described in Chapter 2. While most people know they have excess body fat (at least in certain areas), others may be surprised to learn that their body composition is less than ideal — that the weight scale has not told them the whole story. Optimal body fat percentage should not exceed 20% for women or 15% for men.

Unfortunately, a large segment of the American population is obese. Obesity is one of the major health problems in the United States today. The average American gains one pound of weight each year beyond the age of 25, and this gain is in the form of fat! Furthermore, we know there is a high relationship between obesity and increased risk of death from a variety of diseases. Studies show that obesity may not only increase the risk of developing some diseases but may aggravate diseases which are caused by other factors. Specifically, obesity has been linked to the following problems:

1. High blood pressure.
2. Increased level of cholesterol and triglycerides.
3. Bone and joint disorders.
4. Diabetes.
5. Lower back difficulties.
6. Respiratory ailments.
7. Higher incidence of accidents, surgical and pregnancy complications.

There is little doubt that obesity is a threat to the quality and possibly the length of one's life.

The Causes of Obesity

Do you know how obesity develops? What are the major causes of obesity? Heredity? Environment? Emotional problems? Lack of activity? Obviously, the answer may vary from individual to individual, and it is likely that more than one cause is involved.

To begin with, we must recognize the role heredity plays. Some individuals are born with more of a tendency to become obese. Reasons for this include: (1) an abnormal carbohydrate metabolism; (2) an abnormally efficient fat-storing mechanism; (3) physiological traits which are passed on genetically; and (4) an unusually high number of fat cells. However, even if there is some genetic tendency to become obese, it is not inevitable. We can control and prevent it!

Our environment may be another cause of obesity due to acquired family eating habits or culturally developed attitudes toward weight. Eating patterns which contribute to obesity are typically established early in life. Overeating by young children tends to increase the number of fat cells and contribute to the problem of controlling weight during adulthood. Since eating habits are established early in life, overfeeding children can be the cause for future weight problems.

Another reason cited for obesity is emotional overeating—the situation in which one turns to food to relieve stress or anxiety. Some individuals use food when they are angry, depressed, bored, frustrated, nervous, or upset. Anyone caught in this pattern needs to recognize the situation and identify behavior modification methods which can help solve the problem.

Another factor to consider is that the basal metabolism rate differs among people. The basal metabolism rate is the rate at which the body uses energy to maintain itself while at complete rest, and it declines gradually as one grows older. This rate drops when we sleep, is generally higher in men, and increases as a result of exercise. Therefore, although each of us is different, we do have some means of increasing our basal metabolism rate.

Jean Mayer, a leading authority on nutrition, states that inactivity is the most important reason for the high incidence of obesity in Western societies. Our sedentary lifestyle has been the major cause of the problem — not overeating. As a matter of fact, it appears that the majority of obese individuals do not eat any more than the non-obese. Clearly, sedentary lifestyles have contributed to the high incidence of obesity. We simply do not have a level of activity that will "burn up" the calories we take in each day. Therefore, the real key to controlling obesity is regular exercise. We must include a planned exercise program as part of our daily lives.

The Calorie

Since the basic principle of weight control depends on the ratio between caloric intake and caloric expenditure, we need to understand what a calorie is and how many we actually need. The calorie is the common unit of measurement used to express the potential energy of food. Calories are actually by-products of the chemical changes which our bodies produce from the food we eat. We derive calories or energy from fat (9 calories per gram), carbohydrates (4 calories per gram), and protein (4 calories per gram). From these various caloric sources we obtain the energy needed to digest food, conduct our activities, and maintain body heat. The basic energy needs of the body are based on size, age, and type and amount of daily physical activity. If the food we eat provides us with a surplus of calories — more than we can use at the moment — our body has the ability to store these calories for use in the form of fat. One pound of fat is equivalent to 3,500 excess calories.

Determining the precise number of calories required to maintain your ideal weight is not a simple matter; however, you can determine the approximate number of calories needed per day:

1. Multiply your **ideal** weight by 10 (this determines the number of calories you use at rest — basal metabolic rate or BMR).

2. Based on your level of activity, add one of the following: sedentary — add 1/3 again of your BMR; moderately active (90 minutes of exercise per week)— add 1/2 again your BMR; very active (jog or run 5 miles a day)—may double your BMR (11).

Men generally have a higher minimum caloric need than women, because of a greater proportion of musculature, less fat, and larger size. More energy is required to transform food to energy when more muscle tissue is present .

By calculating the number of calories consumed in our diets and the number expended through the BMR and our daily activities, we can

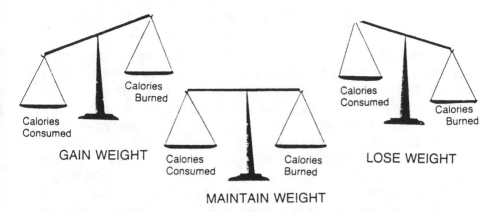

GAIN WEIGHT

Calories Burned

Calories Consumed

MAINTAIN WEIGHT

Calories Consumed

Calories Burned

LOSE WEIGHT

Calories Consumed

Calories Burned

determine if caloric balance has been achieved. The diagram above reflects the importance of analyzing caloric intake and expenditure if one is to achieve and maintain the correct weight.

Caloric Expenditure

When a person has an inactive lifestyle, it is very easy for caloric intake to exceed the energy demands of the body and therefore result in the accumulation of fat deposits. Some people are of the opinion that increasing the exercise level will lead to a corresponding increase in appetite; however, such is not the case. Most studies show that increased activity may stimulate increased food intake but it does not increase above the required energy expenditure. Vigorous, aerobic exercise sustained for an adequate duration will actually cause the body to use fat as a fuel source.

During exercise caloric expenditure can be calculated by measuring the amount of oxygen used in performing the activity. Energy expenditures for different activities vary according to body weight and skill level. Approximations have been prepared from actual measurements and are listed in Appendix H. Generally speaking, exercising with more intensity in a given activity does not increase the caloric expenditure as much as exercising longer and/or covering more distance (12).

Fad Diets

Fad diets are extremely popular because everyone is looking for a quick easy way to achieve weight control. However, fad dieting ultimately leads to failure because it usually does not result in a permanent weight loss. The main shortcoming of fad diets is that they do not bring about a change in basic eating habits and lifestyle. Losing weight is not a temporary, short term problem, so "going on" a diet (and, of course, eventually "going off it") will not solve the problem. To be effective, a diet must be considered from a long-range view. Permanent eating habits that will lead not only to weight management but to a healthy life must be established. Therefore, the best strategy for a lifetime of successful weight control is a sound, nutritious diet combined with regular, vigorous exercise.

Actually it is fortunate that so few people can stay on a fad diet. Most quick reducing diets lack the necessary nutritional balance and may cause great harm if adhered to for long periods of time. In addition, fad diets tend to disturb the body's metabolic balance and returning to "normal" is difficult. This may cause the individual to deposit more fat than usual after going off the diet. Some diets even make the claim that they provide a special metabolic combination of foods which accelerates weight loss. There is no such magic combination just as no one food can help break down fat. Also, remember there is no such thing as a "fattening food" — it is the total number of calories in all foods eaten that determines whether you gain weight. Fat deposits can result from excess calories from any source — carbohydrates, proteins, and alcohol, as well as fats.

Fasting

Some people mistakenly seek semi-starvation or fasting as a means of quick weight loss. The weight loss experienced with fasting and other drastic measures is mainly lean body mass or muscle. Fasting tends to confuse the body and it starts burning up the wrong tissues. Research clearly shows that when fasting only one-third of the weight loss is fatty tissue, while two-thirds is lean body tissue. The reason for this occurrence is that when energy intake is too low, the body maintains the blood glucose level by converting the available amino acids in muscle tissue to glucose.

Another problem arising from extreme caloric deprivation is that the body decreases its metabolic rate. Therefore, calories are burned more slowly and even an extremely small number of calories are sufficient to maintain one's weight. This also triggers the mechanism which causes the body to store fat more efficiently, thus a decrease in lean muscle tissue and an increase in fat storage, to say nothing of the potential health problems which an individual can suffer through a prolonged or consistent program of fasting. Fasting is certainly not recommended as an approach to effective and safe weight loss.

Diet Aids (Pills, Candy, Gum, Etc.)

The basic problem with all diet aids is similar to that of fad diets — they do not meet the nutritional needs of the individual and they do not bring about a change in the basic eating habits of the individual. The goals of such aids are to curb the appetite, numb the taste buds, or provide a feeling of fullness. Most pills contain a drug called phenylpropanolamine (PPA) which your body can build a tolerance to and which can lead to psychological dependence. Some pills have caffeine to relieve the feeling of fatigue or diuretics which cause only water weight loss. The chewing gum or candy-type diet aids depend on benzocaine, a mild topical anesthetic, to numb your taste buds.

Just because a diet aid is sold over the counter doesn't mean it is completely safe. Certain individuals may be susceptible to a particular chemical, and unintentionally overdose on a drug which is found in other medications being taken, and some may develop other side effects. Obviously, however, the major drawback is that such an approach does not contribute to a permanent weight loss.

GUIDELINES FOR PERMANENT WEIGHT CONTROL

As stated previously, permanent weight control is most effectively achieved through a program of sound nutrition and regular exercise. The goal is to develop a habit of good eating and activity that is part of our lives. Basic guidelines which should be considered in establishing a program for permanent weight control are as follows:

1. The program should be based on an analysis of current eating and exercise habits so that specific modifications in lifestyle can be adapted which will be maintained throughout life. The program should fit your lifestyle.

2. For effective weight loss the total calorie intake should be less than the total calories "burned" (negative caloric balance).

3. The diet should contain the percentage of required nutrients established for an optimal diet (see Chapter 9).

4. Weight loss will generally be more lasting if it is gradual. A safe recommendation is to lose no more than two to three pounds per week unless under a doctor's supervision.

5. A regular exercise program should be developed to maximize the calorie expenditure and the loss of fat tissue.

6. Try to select foods providing the highest food value and the fewest calories; i.e., high in vitamins and minerals but low in fat. Make the most of the calories included in your diet.

7. Avoid trying fad diets or "quick" weight loss programs that may be worthless and dangerous.

8. Attempt to balance your caloric intake throughout the day rather than in one or two heavy meals.

9. Remember that your weight loss may not follow a steady rate. Your body may make changes and adjustments that could lead you to believe your diet is not working. So don't be discouraged.

10. Caloric intake of fewer than 1500 calories per day for men and 1200 calories per day for women is not recommended as safe over long periods of time.

11. Avoid getting bored by selecting from a variety of foods.

12. One approach to a successful weight management program is to establish a system of food trade-offs or substitutes. The list below gives you an idea of how this approach can help you enjoy delicious foods and avoid extra calories.

Calorie Saving Ideas

Instead of:	Try:	Calories Saved:
1 oz. bag potato chips	1 cup plain popcorn	120
1 cup whole milk	1 cup 1% lowfat milk	45
1/2 cup ice cream	1/2 cup ice milk	45
3 oz. French fries	3 oz. baked potato	190
1/4 cup sour cream	1/4 cup plain lowfat yogurt	55
1/12 frosted layer cake	1/12 angel food cake	185
3 oz. prime rib	3 oz. lean meat (eye of round)	140
1/2 chicken breast, fried	1/2 chicken breast, baked	175
1 bagel, 1 oz. cream cheese	1 bagel, 1 oz. cottage cheese	80
2 cups fettuccine Alfredo	2 cups spagetti, tomato sauce	350
1/2 cup potato salad	1 cup raw vegetable salad	140
2 T bottled French dressing	2 T low-calorie French dressing	150
1 Danish pastry	half an English muffin	150
7 oz. Tom Collins	6 oz. wine cooler with soda	150
1 cup sugar-coated cornflakes	1 cup plain corn flakes	60
1/2 cup pineapple chunks in heavy syrup	1/2 cup pineapple chunks in juice	25

Analyzing Your Caloric Needs

A basic approach to improving your diet and establishing a method of weight control is to analyze your caloric intake and expenditure. It is important to remove all guesswork from the process, and base your decisions on accurate knowledge of your specific needs.

Most people have a very inaccurate concept of their caloric intake. Even those who appear to be calorie conscious need to keep specific records to maintain accuracy. Therefore, the first recommendation is to collect information about your daily food intake. Lab 8 will assist you in gathering the needed information and help you recognize the patterns, problems, and possible solutions to improving your diet plan. Although time-consuming, this project reveals important information needed for assistance in establishing a long-term approach to permanent weight control.

The next step is to analyze your caloric expenditure. Lab 8 in the Appendix will enable you to calculate your current calorie needs as well as identify future exercise programs to increase this expenditure. By knowing your caloric needs, by carefully analyzing your daily food intake, and by determining your potential caloric expenditure, you can achieve your goal more quickly without the risk of jeopardizing your overall health. It may not be easy and it may require some sacrifices on your part, but if you really make the commitment the results are sure.

QUESTIONS AND ANSWERS

Can I spot reduce?

It is now very clear that one *cannot* spot reduce. Exercising the muscles in a particular area will not cause the fat around that muscle to be broken down for energy. During vigorous exercise the muscles call upon fat storage deposits throughout the body for fuel. Heredity determines our particular distribution of fat deposits. That is the reason each of us gains weight in different areas. The best way to lose fat is to participate in vigorous activity that can be sustained for long periods of time.

How does exercise contribute to weight control?

Exercise can play an important role in your effort to regulate weight. Not only does the exercise burn calories, it also helps maintain muscle tone. An added benefit can be improvement in the body's ability to burn fat. Vigorous exercise over a period of time enables the body to more efficiently use its stores of fat as muscle fuel.

SUGGESTED LABS

Lab 9   Weight Control Contract

REFERENCES

1. Allsen, P., Harrison , J., and Vance, B. *Fitness for Life.* Wm. C. Brown Co., Dubuque, Iowa, 1984.
2. Cotterman, Sandra. *Y's Way to Weight Management.* Human Kinetics Publishers, Champaign, Illinois, 1985.
3. Dusek, Dorothy. *Thin and Fit: Your Personal Lifestyle.* Wadsworth Publishing Co., Belmont, California, 1982.
4. Fisher, A.Garth and Conlee, Robert K. *The Complete Book of Physical Fitness.* Brigham Young University Press, Provo, Utah, 1979.
5. Garrison, L., Leslie, P., and Blackmore, D. *Fitness and Figure Control.* Mayfield Publishing Co., Palo Alto, California, 1981.
6. Garrison, Linda and Reed, Ann. *Fitness for Every Body.* Mayfield Publishing Co., Palo Alto, California, 1980.
7. Getchell, Bud. *The Fitness Book.* Benchmark Press, Inc., Indianapolis, 1987.
8. Getchell, Bud. *Physical Fitness: A Way of Life.* John Wiley & Sons, New York, 1983.
9. Hockey, Robert V. *Physical Fitness — The Pathway to Healthful Living.* C.V. Mosby Co., St. Louis, 1985.
10. Lindsey, R., Jones, B., and Whitley, A. *Body Mechanics.* Wm. C. Brown Co., Dubuque, Iowa, 1979.
11. Miller, David and Allen, Earl. *Fitness: A Lifetime Commitment.* Burgess Publishing Co., Minneapolis, 1986.
12. Sharkey, Brian. *Physiology of Fitness.* Human Kinetics Pubishers, Champaign, Illinois, 1979.
13. U.S. Dept. of Health and Human Services. *Exercise and Your Heart.*, U.S. Government Printing Office, Washington, 1981.

Chapter Eleven

Completing the Picture
A PLAN FOR STRESS REDUCTION

We all live with many different kinds of stress. Stress and anxiety are a part of everyday living. Hans Selye, pioneer in the study of stress, describes stress as a non-specific psychological response to anything that challenges the body (10). These responses can be either physical or emotional. Physical responses to stress include an increase in blood pressure, heart rate, respiratory rate, and muscle tension. Emotional responses to stress include, fear, anxiety, and depression.

Positive stress is referred to as eustress and is a contributor to self-esteem, an important ingredient associated with success. Many very accomplished people attribute their success to the motivating effect of the stress they experience on their jobs. According to Dr. Suzanne Kobasa, psychologist at the University of Chicago, certain people seem to be particularly able to handle stress without it affecting their health, no matter how intense their job pressures or family responsibilities. Recent studies have shown that stress can be a crucial and productive part of everyday life. An individual with a healthy attitude about his/her life can channel stress into a positive experience.

STRESSORS

Stressors are physical, social or psychological events that trigger a stress reaction. Some stressors are clearly identified, such as a failing grade, or an angry parent, while emotional stressors like unhappiness or depression are not so easily identified (4) .

Negative stress or distress can cause serious health problems by lowering the body's resistance to disease. Some common examples of distressors associated with daily life include: financial problems, overcrowding,occupational distress, academic failure, and family problems. Most people will experience one or more of these distressors in their lifetime. A way to cope is to recognize them and understand your reactions to them. Smoking, overeating, overworking, or arguing are not positive ways in which to deal with distress. The following diseases and conditions have been identified with stressful lifestyles (4):

Cardiovascular Disease: coronary artery disease, pains in the chest, hypertension.

Muscle-related Disorders: clenching of the teeth, shoulder and backaches, tension headaches.

Allergic Disease: colds or swelling, hayfever, asthma.

Oral Conditions: thumb sucking, nail biting, tooth decay, cold sores.

If you recognize any of the symptoms, it may be time to develop some coping techniques to deal with stress-relates problems. Listen to your body, build your strength and mental courage, organize your time and learn how to relax your mind and your body.

THE BODY'S RESPONSE TO STRESS

(Adapted from Core Concepts in Health *by Insel and Roth,*
Mayfield Publishing Co., 1988)

Endophins are released.

The hearing becomes more acute.

The rate of breathing is accelerated by the heart and strength of contraction is increased.

Digestion stops.

More red blood corpuscles are released by spleen.

Secretion of epinephrine and norepinephrine is stimulated by the adrenal glands, increasing blood sugar, blood pressure, and heart rate; also causing an increase in amount of fat in the blood.

Secretions by pancreas decrease.

Intestinal muscles loosen.

Contraction of voluntary (skeletal) muscles throughout the body.

The pupils of the eye dilate, admitting more light to increase vision sensitivity.

The mucous membranes of throat and nose shrink; muscles force wider opening of passages so that air may flow through more easily.

Saliva and mucous secretion decreases.

More air is allowed into lungs as bronchi dilates.

In order to flush out waste and cool overheating system by evaporation, perspiration increases, particularly in armpits, groin, hands, and feet.

Liver releases sugar into the bloodstream in order to provide energy for brain and muscles.

Skin contracts, producing goose pimples.

Blood vessels dilate in the external genitals.

Blood vessels contract in the skin, brain, viscera, and skeletal muscles.

More white corpuscles are produced by bone marrow throughout the body.

EUSTRESS

Eustress, the stressors that have positive effects on our lives, include events like graduation from college, beginning a new career, getting married, or becoming physically fit. Eustress includes more than events in life, it can be feelings of success and self-confidence.

Three personality traits that have been identified with those who most often experience eustress are (8):
1. Commitment — a dedication to self, work, family, and other important values
2. Control — a sense of personal control over one's life
3. Challenge — the ability to see change in one's life as a challenge to conquer

Any bad stress can be turned into a positive force in your life. The main objective is to get your life in control when times become overly stressful.

Stress and the College Student

College related stress is usually the result of pressure to succeed. For many, the reality of being away from home and independent is very threatening. The need to make friends and feel comfortable in a new environment can also be stressful. Large classes and the feeling of anonymity may be intimidating for a freshman whereas competing with younger, "brighter" students might be threatening to an older student returning to school. If you experience any of the following symptoms, you might be distressed and need to utilize relaxation activities.
- loss of energy
- loss of motivation
- oversleeping or insomnia
- overeating or loss of appetite
- inability to concentrate
- low output of quality work

TECHNIQUES FOR STRESS MANAGEMENT

Healthy stress management means developing positive attitudes about dealing with present and future stressors. Self-esteem and self-confidence help you cope with stressors. You must learn to develop the self-communication skills necessary for managing stressful situations when they occur. Rather than viewing stressors as adversaries, we should learn to view them as exercises in life (9).

Aerobic Exercise and Stress

According to Dr. Kenneth Cooper, the pioneer and originator of the aerobic concept, we deal with stress at two levels(2):
1. Specific stress situations that occur during the course of an ordinary day.
2. Our ability to relieve ourselves of the stress at the end of an especially pressure-filled day, so that we are more relaxed and energized and capable of enjoying the events of the evening.

Numerous studies have suggested that aerobic exercise has a positive effect on controlling anxiety reactions. It has been observed that the heart rates of individuals change when they move from a low-pressure, low-anxiety state to a highly stressful situation.

Included among the many benefits of aerobic exercise is a lowered resting heart rate. The reason for the lower resting heart rate is twofold.

1. Being aerobically fit causes a slight increase in the size of the heart making it stronger and more efficient. This results in a greater amount of blood being pumped per beat which means the heart beats fewer times per minute.

2. When the resting heart rate decreases in an aerobically fit individual, it tends to stay down under stressful conditions that might ordinarily elevate it.

A lowered heart rate during stressful situations helps you stay calm and in control of your emotions.

Stress, fear and intense emotions causes the adrenal glands to respond by secreting adrenaline into the circulatory system causing the heart to beat faster. Unfortunately, in our relatively sedentary society, this response could be counterproductive if it stressed a poorly conditioned person's heart beyond its capacity.

Researchers are finding that the timing of aerobic exercise can also be a factor in controlling stress. If you exercise at the end of a very stressful day, aerobic activity can help you dissipate stress by removing the accumulated adrenal secretions from a tension-filled day. Exercise acts as nature's waste removal process and helps the body return to a more relaxed, balanced state.

METHODS OF STRESS MANAGEMENT

1. **Aerobic Exercise.** Getting involved in physical activity helps alleviate stress and supports the emotional strategies that are a part of stress management.

2. **Relaxation Techniques**

   Deep Breathing. Close your eyes and focus on a single object. Breathe in through your nose and mouth, hold your breath, and slowly exhale for a count of three. Repeat until you feel comfortable and relaxed.

   Deep Muscle Relaxation. Using this technique you alternately tense, then relax the muscles of the face, neck, shoulders and back.

   Meditation involves deep breathing and is a mental exercise used to gain control of yourself. Meditation techniques can be learned individually in a class or workshop. A trained instructor provides a secret word or sound that you repeat and the repetition helps prevent distracting thoughts from entering your mind.

3. **Biofeedback.** This method is used to control heart rate, blood pressure, and skin temperature or to relax certain muscle groups. A monitoring device emits a sound when changes occur in the body. Biofeedback training requires special equipment and a trained professional.

4. **Proper Nutrition.** Avoid high calorie snacks and calorie-laden meals. Limit the amount of caffeinated beverages you drink and substitute sugary snacks with fruit, sparkling water, breads, and muffins.

5. **Adequate Rest.** Be sure to get the amount of sleep necessary for you to rehabilitate your body. This is best accomplished by developing a routine of going to sleep at approximately the same time every evening.

6. **Support Groups.** Friends, family members and coworkers are people who can provide emotional and psychological support. Talk to a good friend at least once a day and share the good and bad events of your life. Also, participate in community activities and get involved with life.

Stress is here to stay. Our lives will never be stress free, there is no perfect job, no perfect relationship, and no perfect body; however, there is an almost perfect solution to stress management and that is **exercise!**

QUESTIONS AND ANSWERS

What are some of the common symptoms associated with stress?

Headaches, backaches, and tension in the neck and shoulders are some common symptoms.

What is "burnout"?

Burnout is a state of mental and physical exhaustion resulting often-times from frustration and too much stress. Individuals who feel little control over their lives or their jobs often experience burnout.

Frequently the terms "Type A" personality and "Type B" personality are used to describe how different individuals deal with stress. What do these descriptions mean?

A "Type A" personality defines those people who have the "hurry-up syndrome" that usually leads to cardiovascular problems. "Type B" personality is more relaxed and laid back and less likely to suffer from stress and burnout. A third category, "Type C," is a combination of the two in that they channel their stress and energies into positive directions.

Is all stress bad for you?

No. Eustress, a positive stress, provides opportunities for personal growth and development.

What can I do to minimize stressful situations in my life?

First, set realistic and manageable goals for yourself. You may have unrealistic expectations of yourself and others.

What is the best and most productive way of dealing with stress?

The answer to this question may vary from person to person. There are many ways to deal with stress, a good aerobics program is an excellent way to resist stressors and cope with stress-related situations.

Are there any things that contribute to stress and stress related situations?

Yes. Foods and drugs affect stress management. Foods high in fats, sugars, and salts can influence your mood and physical health. Caffeine, nicotine, alcohol and over-the-counter drugs can also have a negative effect on your stress management.

SUGGESTED LABS

Lab 15   Stress Assessment

REFERENCES

1. Cooper, K.H." Coping with Stress," *Aerobic News* 3(1) 1, 1988.
2. Cooper, K.H. *The Aerobics Program for Total Well-Being.* Bantam Books, Toronto, 1982.
3. Corbin, C.B. and Lindsey, R. *Concepts of Physical Fitness with Laboratories.* Wm. C. Brown Co., Dubuque, Iowa,1988.
4. Donatelle, R., Davis, L.C. and Hoover, C.F. *Access to Health.* Prentice Hall, Englewood Cliffs, New Jersey, 1988.
5. Eliot, R.S. "Are You a Hot Reactor?" *Shape* 6(6)66-73, 1987.
6. Friedman, M. and Roseman, R.H. *Type A Behavior and Your Heart.* Knopf Publishers, New York, 1974.
7. Girdano, D.A. and Everly, G.S. *Controlling Stress and Tension: A Holistic Approach.* Prentice Hall, Englewood Cliffs, New Jersey, 1986.
8. Kobasa, S.O. "How Much Stress Can You Survive?" *Annual Editions of Health.* Duskin Publishers, Gilford, Connecticut,1987/88.
9. Selinger S. "Stress Can Be Good for You." *Annual Editions of Health.* Duskin Publishers, Gilford, Connecticut,1987/88.
10. Selye, H. *The Stress of Life.* McGraw-Hill, New York, 1956. Englewood Cliffs, New Jersey, !986.

APPENDICES

APPENDIX A. ANALYSIS OF BODY FAT

Described below are the techniques used in obtaining skin fold measurements and diagrams of the specific location of the measurements. By taking the sum of measurements for various sites one can predict the percent of body fat. Individual values at the sites may be used to note changes in body composition that occur.

Directions for taking measurement:

1. All measurements should be taken from the right side of the body.

2. Measurements should be taken prior to exercise since sweating and increased blood flow make measurement more difficult.

3. Three measurements of each area should be taken to assure accuracy.

4. The calipers must be placed next to the thumb and index finger and allowed to close completely before the measurement is recorded.

Location of measurements:

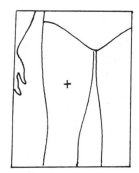

Thigh

A vertical fold midway between the groin line and the patella.

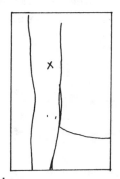

Tricep

A vertical fold midway between the shoulder and elbow joints.

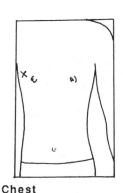

Chest

A diagonal fold between the armpit and nipple.

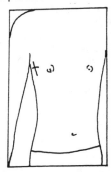

Axilla

A vertical fold on the side at nipple level.

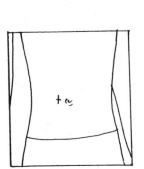

Abdominal

A vertical fold approximately one inch to the right of the navel.

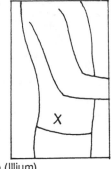

Hip (Illium)

A diagonal fold just above the crest of the hip bone.

BODY COMPOSITION RATING SCALE
Skinfolds
Norms — Males 35 Years and Younger

Rating	Percent Fat	Chest mm	Abdomen mm	Ilium mm	Axilla mm
Very Lean	6	3	4	4	4
Lean	9	7	8	6	8
Leaner Than Ave.	14	12	16	11	13
Average	18	15	21	16	17
Fatter Than Ave.	22	18	27	20	21
Fat	25	22	34	26	25
Very Fat	30	28	44	33	33

Norms — Males 36-45 Years Old

Rating	Percent Fat	Chest mm	Abdomen mm	Ilium mm	Axilla mm
Very Lean	8	4	6	4	4
Lean	10	8	10	8	10
Leaner Than Ave.	15	13	17	13	15
Average	19	16	22	17	19
Fatter Than Ave.	23	19	28	22	23
Fat	27	24	35	28	28
Very Fat	32	30	45	37	35

Norms — Males 46 Years and Older

Rating	Percent Fat	Chest mm	Abdomen mm	Ilium mm	Axilla mm
Very Lean	9	5	6	6	6
Lean	11	8	11	9	11
Leaner Than Ave.	16	14	18	15	17
Average	21	17	23	19	21
Fatter Than Ave.	24	20	29	23	24
Fat	29	24	36	30	30
Very Fat	34	31	46	39	36

Source: Y's Way To Physical Fitness

BODY COMPOSITION RATING SCALE

Norms — Females 35 Years and Younger

Rating	Percent Fat	Tricep mm	Abdomen mm	Ilium mm
Very Lean	9	5	5	4
Lean	14	7	8	7
Leaner Than Ave.	18	12	14	13
Average	22	15	19	16
Fatter Than Ave.	24	19	25	20
Fat	28	25	33	29
Very Fat	35	30	40	35

Norms — Females 36-45 Years

Rating	Percent Fat	Tricep mm	Abdomen mm	Ilium mm
Very Lean	10	6	6	5
Lean	16	9	8	8
Leaner Than Ave.	20	13	14	14
Average	23	17	19	18
Fatter Than Ave.	26	21	25	21
Fat	31	26	33	29
Very Fat	37	32	40	37

Norms — Females 46 Years and Older

Rating	Percent Fat	Tricep mm	Abdomen mm	Ilium mm
Very Lean	11	8	8	7
Lean	18	10	10	9
Leaner Than Ave.	21	15	15	16
Average	25	18	20	18
Fatter Than Ave.	30	23	26	22
Fat	34	27	35	32
Very Fat	41	34	43	39

Source: Y's Way To Physical Fitness

PERCENT FAT ESTIMATES FOR MEN

Sum of Four Skinfolds

Chest, Ilium, Abdomen, Axilla

Sum of 4 Skinfolds	Age To Last Year								
	18 to 22	23 to 27	28 to 32	33 to 37	38 to 42	43 to 47	48 to 52	53 to 57	58 and older
8-12	1.9	2.5	3.2	3.8	4.4	5.0	5.7	6.3	6.9
13-17	3.3	3.9	4.5	5.1	5.7	6.4	7.0	7.6	8.2
18-22	4.5	5.2	5.8	6.4	7.0	7.7	8.3	8.9	9.5
23-27	5.8	6.4	7.1	7.7	8.3	8.9	9.5	10.2	10.8
28-32	7.1	7.7	8.3	8.9	9.5	10.2	10.8	11.4	12.0
33-37	8.3	8.9	9.5	10.1	10.8	11.4	12.0	12.6	13.2
38-42	9.5	10.1	10.7	11.3	11.9	12.6	13.2	13.8	14.4
43-47	10.6	11.3	11.9	12.5	13.1	13.7	14.4	15.0	15.6
48-52	11.8	12.4	13.0	13.6	14.2	14.9	15.5	16.1	16.7
53-57	12.9	13.5	14.1	14.7	15.4	16.0	16.6	17.2	17.9
58-62	14.0	14.6	15.2	15.8	16.4	17.1	17.7	18.3	18.9
63-67	15.0	15.6	16.3	16.9	17.5	18.1	18.8	19.4	20.0
68-72	16.1	16.7	17.3	17.9	18.5	19.2	19.8	20.4	21.0
73-77	17.1	17.7	18.3	18.9	19.5	20.2	20.8	21.4	22.0
78-82	18.0	18.7	19.3	19.9	20.5	21.0	21.8	22.4	23.0
83-87	19.0	19.6	20.2	20.8	21.5	22.1	22.7	23.3	24.0
88-92	19.9	20.5	21.2	21.8	22.4	23.0	23.6	24.3	24.9
93-97	20.8	21.4	22.1	22.7	23.3	23.9	24.5	25.2	25.8
98-102	21.7	22.3	22.9	23.5	24.2	24.8	25.4	26.0	26.7
103-107	22.5	23.2	23.8	24.4	25.0	25.6	26.3	26.9	27.5
108-112	23.4	24.0	24.6	25.2	25.8	26.5	27.1	27.7	28.3
113-117	24.1	24.8	25.4	26.0	26.6	27.3	27.9	28.5	29.1
118-122	24.9	25.5	26.2	26.8	27.4	28.0	28.6	29.3	29.9
123-127	25.7	26.3	26.9	27.5	28.1	28.8	29.4	30.0	30.6
128-132	26.4	27.0	27.6	28.2	28.8	29.5	30.1	30.7	31.3
133-137	27.1	27.7	28.3	28.9	29.5	30.2	30.8	31.4	32.0
138-142	27.7	28.3	29.0	29.6	30.2	30.8	31.4	32.1	32.7
143-147	28.3	29.0	29.6	30.2	30.8	31.5	32.1	32.7	33.3
148-152	29.0	29.6	30.2	30.8	31.4	32.1	32.7	33.3	33.9
153-157	29.5	30.2	30.8	31.4	32.0	32.7	33.3	33.9	34.5
158-162	30.1	30.7	31.3	31.9	32.6	33.2	33.8	34.4	35.1
163-167	30.6	31.2	31.9	32.5	33.1	33.7	34.3	35.0	35.6
168-172	31.1	31.7	32.4	33.0	33.6	34.2	34.8	35.5	36.1
173-177	31.6	32.2	32.8	33.5	34.1	34.7	35.3	35.9	36.6
178-182	32.0	32.7	33.3	33.9	34.5	35.2	35.8	36.4	37.0
183-187	32.5	33.1	33.7	34.3	34.9	35.6	36.2	26.8	37.4
188-192	32.9	33.5	34.1	34.7	35.3	36.0	36.6	37.2	37.8
193-197	33.2	33.8	34.5	35.1	35.7	36.3	37.0	36.8	38.2
198-202	33.6	34.2	34.8	35.4	36.1	36.7	37.3	37.9	38.5
203-207	33.9	34.5	35.1	35.7	36.4	37.0	37.6	38.2	38.9

Source: Y's Way To Physical Fitness

PERCENT FAT ESTIMATE FOR WOMEN

Sum of Three Skinfolds

Triceps, Abdomen, Ilium

Sum of 3 Skinfolds	Age to Last Year								
	18 to 22	23 to 27	28 to 32	33 to 37	38 to 42	43 to 47	48 to 52	53 to 57	58 and older
8-12	8.8	9.0	9.2	9.4	9.5	9.7	9.9	10.1	10.3
13-17	10.8	10.9	11.1	11.3	11.5	11.7	11.8	12.0	12.2
18-22	12.6	12.8	13.0	13.2	13.4	13.5	13.7	13.9	14.1
23-27	14.5	14.6	14.8	15.0	15.2	15.4	15.6	15.7	15.9
28-32	16.2	16.4	16.6	16.8	17.0	17.1	17.3	17.5	17.7
33-37	17.9	18.1	18.3	18.5	18.7	18.9	19.0	19.2	19.4
38-42	19.6	19.8	20.0	20.2	20.3	20.5	20.7	20.9	21.1
43-47	21.2	21.4	21.6	21.8	21.9	22.1	22.3	22.5	22.7
48-52	22.8	22.9	23.1	23.3	23.5	23.7	23.8	24.0	24.2
53-57	24.2	24.4	24.6	24.8	25.0	25.2	25.3	25.5	25.7
									27.1
58-62	25.7	25.9	26.0	26.2	26.4	26.6	26.8	27.0	37.1
63-67	27.1	27.2	27.4	27.6	27.8	28.0	28.2	28.3	28.5
68-72	28.4	28.6	28.7	28.9	29.1	29.3	29.5	29.7	29.8
73-77	29.6	29.8	30.0	30.2	30.4	30.6	30.7	30.9	31.1
78-82	30.9	31.0	31.2	31.4	31.6	31.8	31.9	32.1	32.3
83-87	32.0	32.2	32.4	32.6	32.7	32.9	33.1	33.3	33.5
88-92	33.1	33.3	33.5	33.7	33.8	34.0	34.2	34.4	34.6
93-97	34.1	34.3	34.5	34.7	34.9	35.1	35.2	35.4	35.6
98-102	35.1	35.3	35.5	35.7	35.9	36.0	36.2	36.4	36.6
103-107	36.1	36.2	36.4	36.6	36.8	37.0	37.2	37.3	37.5
108-112	36.9	37.1	37.3	37.5	37.7	37.9	38.0	38.2	38.4
113-117	37.8	37.9	38.1	38.3	39.2	39.4	39.6	39.8	40.0
118-122	38.5	38.7	38.9	39.1	39.4	39.6	39.8	40.0	
123-127	39.2	39.4	39.6	39.8	40.0	40.1	40.3	40.5	40.7
128-132	39.9	40.1	40.2	40.4	40.6	40.8	41.0	41.2	41.3
133-137	40.5	40.7	40.8	41.0	41.2	41.4	41.6	41.7	41.9
138-142	41.0	41.2	41.4	41.6	41.7	41.9	42.1	42.3	42.5
143-147	41.5	41.7	41.9	42.0	42.2	42.4	42.6	42.8	43.0
148-152	41.9	42.1	42.3	42.8	42.6	42.8	43.0	43.2	43.4
153-157	42.3	42.5	42.6	52.8	43.0	43.2	43.4	43.6	43.7
158-162	42.6	42.8	42.0	43.1	43.3	43.5	43.7	43.9	44.1
163-167	42.9	43.0	43.2	43.4	43.6	43.8	44.0	44.1	44.3
168-172	43.1	43.2	43.4	43.6	43.8	44.0	44.2	44.3	44.5
173-177	43.2	43.4	43.6	43.8	43.9	44.1	44.3	44.5	44.7
178-182	43.3	43.5	43.7	43.8	44.0	44.2	44.4	44.6	44.8

APPENDIX B.
NUTRITIONAL ANALYSIS OF SELECTED FAST FOODS

	Calories	Protein (gm)	Carbohydrates (gm)	Fat (gm)	Sodium * (mg)
McDONALD'S					
Egg McMuffin	327	18	26	20	885
Hot Cakes, with Butter and Syrup	472	8	89	9	
Scrambled Eggs	162	12	2	12	
Big Mac	541	26	39	31	1510
Cheeseburger	306	16	31	13	767
Filet O Fish	383	15	34	23	781
French Fries	304	3	26	11	88
Hamburger	257	13	30	9	393
Quarter Pounder	418	26	33	21	735
Apple Pie	300	2	31	19	
Chocolate Shake	364	11	60	9	300
Vanilla Shake	323	10	52	8	
PIZZA HUT					
(1 serving equals one half of a ten inch pizza.)					
Thin 'N Crispy, 1 Serving					
Cheese	450	25	54	15	1386
Pepperoni	430	25	54	15	
Supreme	510	27	51	21	1848
Thick 'N Chewy, 1 Serving					
Cheese	560	34	68	18	
Pepperoni	560	31	68	18	
Supreme	640	36	74	22	
TACO BELL					
Bean Burrito	343	11	48	12	272
Beef Burrito	466	30	37	21	327
Beefy Tostada	291	19	21	15	
Burrito Supreme	457	21	43	22	367
Combination Burrito	404	21	43	16	
Pintos 'N Cheese	168	11	21	5	
Taco	186	15	14	8	
Tostada	179	9	25	6	
BEVERAGES					
Coffee, 6 ounces	2	tr	tr	tr	
Tea, 6 ounces	2	tr	—	tr	
Orange Juice, 6 ounces	82	1	20	tr	
Chocolate Milk, 8 ounces	213	9	28	9	
Skim Milk, 8 ounces	88	9	13	tr	
Whole Milk, 8 ounces	159	9	12	9	
Regular Cola, 8 ounces	96	0	24	0	

* No number in this column means only that the sodium content was not available. It does not mean that the food contains no sodium, since most fast foods contain a very high sodium content.

NUTRITIONAL ANALYSIS OF SELECTED FAST FOODS

	Calories	Protein (gm)	Carbohydrates (gm)	Fat (gm)	Sodium * (mg)
BURGER KING					
Cheeseburger	305	17	29	13	730
Hamburger	252	14	29	9	525
Whopper	660	29	51	32	909
French Fries	314	3	28	10	230
Vanilla Shake	332	11	50	11	
Whaler	584	18	64	46	968
KENTUCKY FRIED CHICKEN					
Individual Pieces(Original Recipe)					
Drumstick	136	14	2	8	760
Breast	241	19	8	15	
Thigh	276	20	12	19	
Wing	151	11	4	10	
DAIRY QUEEN					
Big Brazier Deluxe	470	28	36	24	
Big Brazier Regular	457	27	37	23	
Brazier Dog	273	11	23	15	
Brazier French Fries, 4.0 ounces	320	3	40	16	
Brazier Onion Rings	300	6	33	17	
Fish Sandwich	400	20	41	17	
Banana Split	540	10	91	15	
Buster Bar	390	10	37	22	
Chocolate Dipped Cone, medium	300	7	40	13	
Regular Cone, medium	230	6	35	7	
Dilly Bar	240	4	22	15	
Freeze	520	11	89	13	
Hot Fudge Brownie Delight	570	11	83	22	
LONG JOHN SILVER'S					
Breaded Oysters, 6 pieces	460	14	58	19	
Breaded Clams, 5 ounces	465	13	46	25	
Chicken Planks, 4 pieces	458	27	35	23	
Cole Slaw, 4 ounces	138	1	16	8	
Corn on Cob, 1 piece	174	5	29	4	
Fish with Batter, 2 pieces	318	19	19	19	
French Fries, 3 ounces	320	4	32	15	128
Hush Puppies, 3 pieces	153	1	20	7	
Peg Leg with Batter, 5 pieces	514	25	30	33	
Shrimp with Batter, 6 pieces	269	9	31	13	
Treasure Chest: 2 pieces Fish, 2 Peg Legs	467	25	27	29	1333

* No number in this column means only that the sodium content was not available. It does not mean that the food contains no sodium, since most fast foods contain a very high sodium content.

APPENDIX C. HIDDEN SUGAR (SUCROSE) IN FOODS

Approximate sugar content of popular foods in grams
(5 g = 1 tsp. = 20 calories)

	Food	Serving	Sucrose (grams)
CANDY	Chocolate bar	1 average size	35
	Chocolate cream	1 average size	10
	Chocolate fudge	1½" sq. (15 to 1 lb.)	20
	Chocolate mints	1 medium (20 to 1 lb.)	15
	Marshmallow	1 average (60 to 1 lb.)	7
	Chewing gum	1 stick	3
CAKES AND COOKIES	Chocolate cake	1/12 cake (2 layer icing)	75
	Angel food cake	1/12 of large cake	30
	Sponge cake	1/10 of average cake	30
	Cream puff, iced	1 average custard filled	25
	Doughnut, plain	3" diameter	20
	Macaroons	1 large or 2 small	15
	Gingersnaps	1 medium	5
	Molasses cookies	3½" diameter	10
	Brownies	2" x 2" x ¾"	15
ICE CREAM	Ice cream	⅛ quart (½ cup)	30
	Sherbet	⅛ quart (½ cup)	40
PIE	Apple	1/6 med. pie	60
	Cherry	1/6 med. pie	70
	Raisin	1/6 med. pie	65
	Pumpkin	1/6 med. pie	50
SOFT DRINKS	Sweet carbonated beverage	1 bottle, 6 oz	22
	Ginger ale	6 oz. glass	18
MILK DRINKS	Chocolate	1 cup, 5 oz. milk	30
	Cocoa	1 cup, 5 oz. milk	20
	Eggnog	1 glass, 8 oz. milk	22

	Food	Serving	Sucrose (grams)
SPREADS AND SAUCES	Jam	1 tbs. level	15
	Jelly	1 tbs. level	12
	Marmalade	1 tbs. level	15
	Syrup, maple	1 tbs. level	12
	Honey	1 tbs. level	15
	Chocolate sauce	1 tbs. thick	22
COOKED FRUITS	Peaches, canned in syrup	2 halves, 1 tbs. syrup	18
	Rhubarb, stewed. sweetened	½ cup	40
	Apple sauce. unsweetened	½ cup. scant	10
	Prunes, stewed. sweetened	4 to 5 med. 2 tbs. juice	40
DRIED FRUITS	Apricots, dried	4 to 6 halves	20
	Prunes, dried	3 to 4 medium	20
	Dates, dried	3 to 4 stoned	22
	Figs, dried	1½ to 2 small	20
	Raisins	¼ cup	20
FRUITS AND FRUIT JUICES	Fruit cocktail	½ cup. scant	25
	Orange juice	½ cup. scant	10
	Pineapple juice. unsweetened	½ cup. scant	13
	Grapefruit juice unsweetened	½ cup. scant	11
	Grapefruit, commercial	½ cup. scant	18

SOURCE: Adapted from American Dental Association, Diet and Dental Health. 1967.

APPENDIX D. HIDDEN SALT IN FOODS

Sodium in Processed Foods

Product	Amount	Sodium (mg)
Pepperidge Farm White Bread	2 slices	234
Wonder Enriched Bread	2 slices	355
Pepperidge Farm Whole Wheat Bread	2 slices	214
Kellogg's Corn Flakes	1 ounce	320
Kellogg's Sugar Frosted Flakes	1 ounce	186
Campbell's Tomato Soup	10-ounce serving	1050
Campbell's Tomato Juice	8 ounces	744
Lipton Vegetable Cup-a-Soup	8 ounces	1058
Breakstone's Lowfat Cottage Cheese	½ cup	435
Kraft Processed American Cheese	1 ounce	238
Kraft Cheddar Cheese	1 ounce	190
Morton King Size Turkey Dinner	1 dinner	2567
Swanson Fried Chicken Dinner	1 dinner	1152
Swanson Turkey Dinner	1 dinner	1735
Campbell's Beans & Franks	8 ounces	958
Oscar Mayer Beef Franks	1 frank	425
Chef Boyardee Beefaroni	7.5 ounces	1186
B&M Brick Oven Baked Beans	1 cup	810
Del Monte Whole Green Beans	1 cup	925
McDonald's Big Mac	1	1510
Burger King Whopper	1	909
Arthur Treacher's Fish Sandwich	1	836
Kentucky Fried Chicken Dinner original recipe (3 pieces chicken)	1	2285
Nabisco Premium Saltines	10 (1 ounce)	430
Mister Salty Very Thin Pretzel Sticks	1 ounce	735
Heinz Kosher Dill Pickles	1 large	1137
Heinz Mustard	1 tablespoon	212
Heinz Tomato Ketchup	1 tablespoon	154
Jell-O Chocolate Flavor Instant Pudding & Pie Filling	½ cup	480
Hostess Twinkies	1	190
Pillsbury Chocolate Chip Cookies	3	140
Nabisco Oreo Sandwich Cookies	3	240

Note: Based on analyses by Consumers Union, the Center for Science in the Public Interests, and manufacturers.

Salt in Natural Foods and in Processed Foods

Food	Portion	Sodium content
Salmon, fresh	3 oz.	99 milligrams
Salmon, canned without salt added	3 oz.	41 milligrams
Salmon canned, salt added	3 oz.	443 milligrams
Tuna, canned, low sodium	3 oz.	34 milligrams
Tuna, canned	3 oz.	303 milligrams
Shrimp, fresh	3 oz.	137 milligrams
Shrimp, canned	3 oz.	1,955 milligrams
Swiss cheese	1 oz.	74 milligrams
Swiss cheese style "food"	1 oz.	440 milligrams
Cottage cheese, unsalted	1 oz.	14 milligrams
Cottage cheese, salted	1 oz.	457 milligrams
Beef, lean	3 oz.	55 milligrams
Dried beef, chipped	3 oz.	1,219 milligrams
Frankfurter	1 frank	639 milligrams
Liver	3 oz.	33 milligrams
Braunschweiger	1 slice	324 milligrams
Oatmeal	3/4 cup	1 milligram
Oatmeal, instant, salt added	3/4 cup	283 milligrams
Rice Crispies	1 cup	340 milligrams
Macaroni	1 cup	2 milligrams
Macaroni and beef, canned	1 cup	1,185 milligrams
Beans, lima	1 cup	3 milligrams
Beans, lima, canned	1 cup	465 milligrams
Soy sauce	1 tbsp	1,029 milligrams

APPENDIX E. CALORIES FROM CONDIMENTS

Condiments can fool you — some have as many or more calories than the foods we put them on. Many also are high in fat and therefore should be avoided as much as possible.

Check the list below and see if the calories you are getting are worth it.

Condiment	Calories Per Tbsp.
Vegetable Oil	120
Butter	102
Margarine	102
Mayonnaise	101
Tartar sauce	74
Honey	64
Maple Syrup	60
Jams and Preserves	54
Cream Cheese	52
Sugar	46
Cream (light)	32
Barbecue Sauce	23
Pickle Relish (sweet)	21
Steak sauce	21
Catsup	16
Mustard	15
Worchestershire sauce	12

APPENDIX F. NUTRITIVE VALUES OF FOODS

The following charts are from the publication *Nutritive Value of Foods* published by the United States Department of Agriculture.

Key to Abbreviations

A Item Number (for reference)

B Food, approximate measures, units, and weight
   (edible part unless indicated otherwise in footnotes)

C Water (percent)

D Food energy (calories)

E Protein (grams)

F Fat (grams)

G Fatty Acids: Saturated (total in grams)

H Fatt Acids: Unsaturated — Oleic (grams)

I Fatty Acids: Unsaturated — Linoleic (grams)

J Carbohydrates (grams)

K Calcium (milligrams)

L Phosphorus (milligrams)

M Iron (milligrams)

N Potassium (milligrams)

O Vitamin A value (international units)

P Thiamine (milligrams)

Q Riboflavin (milligrams)

R Niacin (milligrams)

S Ascorbic acid (milligrams)

DAIRY PRODUCTS (CHEESE, CREAM, IMITATION CREAM, MILK, RELATED PRODUCTS)

Butter. See Fats, oils; related products, items 103-108.

(A)	(B)	Grams	(C) Per-cent	(D) Cal-ories	(E) Grams	(F) Grams	(G) Grams	(H) Grams	(I) Grams	(J) Grams	(K) Milli-grams	(L) Milli-grams	(M) Milli-grams	(N) Milli-grams	(O) International units	(P) Milli-grams	(Q) Milli-grams	(R) Milli-grams	(S) Milli-grams
	Cheese:																		
	Natural:																		
1	Blue----- 1 oz	28	42	100	6	8	5.3	1.9	0.2	1	150	110	0.1	73	200	0.01	0.11	0.3	0
2	Camembert (3 wedges per 4-oz container)---- 1 wedge	38	52	115	8	9	5.8	2.2	.2	1	147	132	.1	71	350	.01	.19	.2	0
	Cheddar:																		
3	Cut pieces----- 1 oz	28	37	115	7	9	6.1	2.1	.2	Trace	204	145	.2	28	300	.01	.11	Trace	0
4	Shredded---- 1 cu in	17.2	37	70	4	6	3.7	1.3	.1	Trace	124	68	.1	17	180	Trace	.06	Trace	0
5	Cottage (curd not pressed down) 1 cup	113	37	455	28	37	24.2	8.5	.7	1	815	579	.8	111	1,200	.03	.42	.1	0
	Creamed (cottage cheese, 4% fat):																		
6	Large curd----- 1 cup	225	79	235	28	10	6.4	2.4	.2	6	135	297	.3	190	370	.05	.37	.3	Trace
7	Small curd----- 1 cup	210	79	220	26	9	6.0	2.2	.2	6	126	277	.3	177	340	.04	.34	.3	Trace
8	Low fat (2%)---- 1 cup	226	79	205	31	4	2.8	1.0	.1	8	155	340	.4	217	160	.05	.42	.3	Trace
9	Low fat (1%)---- 1 cup	226	82	165	28	2	1.5	.5	.1	6	138	302	.3	193	80	.05	.37	.2	Trace
10	Uncreamed (cottage cheese dry curd, less than 1/2% fat)---- 1 cup	145	80	125	25	1	.4	.1	Trace	3	46	151	.3	47	40	.04	.21	.2	0
11	Cream----- 1 oz	28	54	100	2	10	6.2	2.4	.2	1	23	30	.3	34	400	Trace	.06	Trace	0
	Mozzarella, made with—																		
12	Whole milk---- 1 oz	28	48	90	6	7	4.4	1.7	.2	1	163	117	.1	21	260	Trace	.08	Trace	0
13	Part skim milk---- 1 oz	28	49	80	8	5	3.1	1.2	.1	1	207	149	.1	27	180	.01	.10	Trace	0
	Parmesan, grated:																		
14	Cup, not pressed down 1 cup	100	18	455	42	30	19.1	7.7	.3	4	1,376	807	1.0	107	700	.05	.39	.3	0
15	Tablespoon---- 1 tbsp	5	18	25	2	2	1.0	.4	Trace	Trace	69	40	Trace	5	40	Trace	.02	Trace	0
16	Ounce---- 1 oz	28	18	130	12	9	5.4	2.2	.1	1	390	229	.3	30	200	.01	.11	Trace	0
17	Provolone---- 1 oz	28	41	100	7	8	4.8	1.7	.1	1	214	141	.1	39	230	.01	.09	Trace	0
	Ricotta, made with—																		
18	Whole milk---- 1 cup	246	72	428	28	32	20.4	7.1	.7	7	509	363	.9	257	1,210	.03	.48	.3	0
19	Part skim milk---- 1 cup	246	74	340	28	19	12.1	4.7	.5	13	669	449	1.1	308	1,060	.05	.46	.2	0
20	Romano---- 1 oz	28	31	110	9	8				1	302	215	Trace	160		.11		0
21	Swiss---- 1 oz	28	37	105	8	8	5.0	1.7	.2	1	272	171	Trace	31	240	.01	.10	Trace	0
	Pasteurized process cheese:																		
22	American---- 1 oz	28	39	105	6	9	5.6	2.1	.2	Trace	174	211	.1	46	340	.01	.10	Trace	0
23	Swiss---- 1 oz	28	42	95	7	7	4.5	1.7	.1	1	219	216	.2	61	230	Trace	.08	Trace	0
24	Pasteurized process cheese food, American---- 1 oz	28	43	95	6	7	4.4	1.7	.1	2	163	130	.2	79	260	.01	.13	Trace	0
25	Pasteurized process cheese spread, American---- 1 oz	28	48	82	5	6	3.8	1.5	.1	2	159	202	.1	69	220	.01	.12	Trace	0
	Cream, sweet:																		
26	Half-and-half (cream and milk)- 1 cup	242	81	315	7	28	17.3	7.0	.6	10	254	230	.2	314	260	.08	.36	.2	2
27	---- 1 tbsp	15	81	20	Trace	2		.4	Trace	1	16	14	Trace	19	20	.01	.02	Trace	Trace
28	Light, coffee, or table 1 cup	240	74	470	6	46	28.8	11.7	1.0	9	231	192	.1	292	1,730	.08	.36	.1	2
29	---- 1 tbsp	15	74	30	Trace	3	1.8	.7	.1	1	14	12	Trace	18	110	Trace	.02	Trace	Trace

No.	Food, approximate measure, and weight (in grams)		Water (%)	Food energy (cal)	Protein (g)	Fat (g)	Saturated (total) (g)	Oleic (g)	Linoleic (g)	Carbohydrate (g)	Calcium (mg)	Phosphorus (mg)	Iron (mg)	Potassium (mg)	Vitamin A (IU)	Thiamin (mg)	Riboflavin (mg)	Niacin (mg)	Ascorbic acid (mg)
	Whipping, unwhipped (volume about double when whipped):																		
30	Light	1 cup	64	700	5	74	46.2	18.3	1.5	7	166	146	.1	231	2,690	0.06	0.30	0.1	Trace
31		1 tbsp	64	45	Trace	5	2.9	1.1	Trace	Trace	10	9	Trace	15	170	Trace	.02	Trace	Trace
32	Heavy	1 cup	58	820	5	88	54.8	22.2	2.0	7	154	149	.1	179	3,500	.05	.26	.1	Trace
33		1 tbsp	58	80	Trace	6	3.5	1.4	.1	Trace	10	9	Trace	11	220	Trace	.02	Trace	Trace
34	Whipped topping, (pressurized)	1 cup	61	155	2	13	8.3	3.4	.3	7	61	54	Trace	88	550	.02	.04	Trace	0
35		1 tbsp	61	10	Trace	1	.4	.2	Trace	Trace	3	3	Trace	4	30	Trace	Trace	Trace	0
36	Cream, sour	1 cup	71	495	7	48	30.0	12.1	1.1	10	268	195	.1	331	1,820	.08	.34	.2	2
37		1 tbsp	71	25	Trace	3	1.6	.6	.1	1	14	10	Trace	17	90	Trace	.02	Trace	Trace
	Cream products, imitation (made with vegetable fat):																		
	Sweet:																		
	Creamers:																		
38	Liquid (frozen)	1 cup	77	335	2	24	22.8	.3	Trace	28	23	157	.1	467	220[2]	0	0	0	0
39		1 tbsp	77	20	Trace	2	1.4	Trace	0	2	1	10	Trace	29	10[2]	0	0	0	0
40	Powdered	1 cup	2	505	5	33	30.6	.9	Trace	52	21	397	Trace	763	190[2]	0	.16[1]	0	0
41		1 tsp	2	10	Trace	1	.7	Trace	0	1	Trace	8	Trace	16	Trace[2]	0	Trace[1]	0	0
	Whipped topping:																		
42	Frozen	1 cup	50	240	1	19	16.3	1.0	.2	17	5	6	.1	14	650[2]	0	0	0	0
43		1 tbsp	50	15	Trace	1	.9	.1	Trace	1	Trace	Trace	Trace	1	30[2]	0	0	0	0
44	Powdered, made with whole milk	1 cup	67	150	3	10	8.5	.6	.1	13	72	69	Trace	121	290[2]	.02	.09	Trace	1
45		1 tbsp	67	10	Trace	Trace	.4	Trace	Trace	1	4	3	Trace	6	10[2]	Trace	Trace	Trace	Trace
46	Pressurized	1 cup	60	185	1	16	13.2	1.4	.2	11	4	13	Trace	13	330[2]	0	0	0	0
47		1 tbsp	60	10	Trace	1	.8	.1	Trace	1	Trace	1	Trace	1	20[2]	0	0	0	0
48	Sour dressing (imitation sour cream) made with nonfat dry milk	1 cup	75	415	8	39	31.2	4.4	1.1	11	266	205	.1	380	20[2]	.09	.38	.2	2
49		1 tbsp	75	20	Trace	2	1.6	.2	.1	1	14	10	Trace	19	Trace[2]	.01	.02	Trace	Trace
	Ice cream. See Milk desserts, frozen (items 75-90).																		
	Ice milk. See Milk desserts, frozen (items 81-93).																		
	Milk:																		
	Fluid:																		
50	Whole (3.3% fat)	1 cup	88	150	8	8	5.1	2.1	.2	11	291	228	.1	370	310[3]	.09	.40	.2	2
51	Lowfat (2%): No milk solids added	1 cup	89	120	8	5	2.9	1.2	.1	12	297	232	.1	377	500	.10	.40	.2	2
52	Milk solids added: Label claim less than 10 g of protein per cup.	1 cup	89	125	9	5	2.9	1.2	.1	12	313	245	.1	397	500	.10	.42	.2	2
53	Label claim 10 or more grams of protein per cup (protein fortified).	1 cup	88	135	10	5	3.0	1.2	.1	14	352	276	.1	447	500	.11	.48	.2	3
54	Lowfat (1%): No milk solids added	1 cup	90	100	8	3	1.6	.7	.1	12	300	235	.1	381	500	.10	.41	.2	2
55	Milk solids added: Label claim less than 10 g of protein per cup.	1 cup	90	105	9	2	1.5	.6	.1	12	313	245	.1	397	500	.10	.42	.2	2
56	Label claim 10 or more grams of protein per cup (protein fortified).	1 cup	89	120	10	3	1.8	.7	.1	14	349	273	.1	444	500	.11	.47	.2	3
57	Nonfat (skim): No milk solids added	1 cup	91	85	8	Trace	.3	.1	Trace	12	302	247	.1	406	500	.09	.37	.2	2

[1]Vitamin A value is largely from beta-carotene used for coloring. Riboflavin value for items 40-41 apply to product with added riboflavin.

[2]Applies to product without added vitamin A. With added vitamin A, value is 500 International Units (I.U.).

DAIRY PRODUCTS (CHEESE, CREAM, IMITATION CREAM, MILK; RELATED PRODUCTS)—Con.

(A)	(B)		Grams	(C) Per-cent	(D) Cal-ories	(E) Grams	(F) Grams	(G) Grams	(H) Grams	(I) Grams	(J) Grams	(K) Milli-grams	(L) Milli-grams	(M) Milli-grams	(N) Milli-grams	(O) Inter-national units	(P) Milli-grams	(Q) Milli-grams	(R) Milli-grams	(S) Milli-grams
	Milk—Continued																			
	Fluid—Continued																			
	Nonfat (skim)—Continued																			
	Milk solids added:																			
58	Label claim less than 10 g of protein per cup.	1 cup	245	90	90	9	1	0.4	0.1	Trace	12	316	255	0.1	418	500	0.10	0.43	0.2	2
59	Label claim 10 or more grams of protein per cup (protein fortified).	1 cup	246	89	100	10	1	.4	.1	Trace	14	352	275	.1	446	500	.11	.48	.2	3
60	Buttermilk	1 cup	245	90	100	8	2	1.3	.5	Trace	12	285	219	.1	371	180	.08	.38	.1	2
	Canned:																			
	Evaporated, unsweetened:																			
61	Whole milk	1 cup	252	74	340	17	19	11.6	5.3	0.4	25	657	510	.5	764	610	.12	.80	.5	5
62	Skim milk	1 cup	255	79	200	19	1	.7	.1	Trace	29	738	497	.7	845	1,000	.11	.79	.4	3
63	Sweetened, condensed	1 cup	306	27	980	24	27	16.8	6.7	.7	166	868	775	.6	1,136	1,000	.28	1.27	.6	8
	Dried:																			
64	Buttermilk	1 cup	120	3	465	41	7	4.3	1.7	.2	59	1,421	1,119	.4	1,910	260	.47	1.90	1.1	7
	Nonfat instant:																			
65	Envelope, net wt., 3.2 oz.	1 envelope	91	4	325	32	1	.4	.1	Trace	47	1,120	896	.3	1,552	2,160	.38	1.59	.8	5
66	Cup	1 cup	68	4	245	24	Trace	.3	.1	Trace	35	837	670	.2	1,160	1,610	.28	1.19	.6	4
	Milk beverages:																			
	Chocolate milk (commercial):																			
67	Regular	1 cup	250	82	210	8	8	5.3	2.2	.2	26	280	251	.6	417	300	.09	.41	.3	2
68	Lowfat (2%)	1 cup	250	84	180	8	5	3.1	1.3	.1	26	284	254	.6	422	500	.10	.42	.3	2
69	Lowfat (1%)	1 cup	250	85	160	8	3	1.5	1.7	.1	26	287	257	.6	426	500	.10	.40	.2	2
70	Eggnog (commercial)	1 cup	254	74	340	10	19	11.3	5.0	.6	34	330	278	.5	420	890	.09	.48	.3	4
71	Malted milk, home-prepared with 1 cup of whole milk and 2 to 3 heaping tsp of malted milk powder (about 3/4 oz): Chocolate	1 cup of milk plus 3/4 oz of powder.	265	81	235	9	9	5.5	—	—	29	304	265	.5	500	330	.14	.43	.7	2
72	Natural	1 cup of milk plus 3/4 oz of powder.	265	81	235	11	10	6.0	—	—	27	347	307	.3	529	380	.20	.54	1.3	2
	Shakes, thick:[8]																			
73	Chocolate, container, net wt., 10.6 oz.	1 container	300	72	355	9	8	5.0	2.0	.2	63	396	378	.9	672	260	.14	.67	.4	0
74	Vanilla, container, net wt., 11 oz.	1 container	313	74	350	12	9	5.9	2.4	.2	56	457	361	.3	572	360	.09	.61	.5	0
	Milk desserts, frozen:																			
	Ice cream:																			
	Regular (about 11% fat):																			
75	Hardened	1/2 gal	1,064	61	2,155	38	115	71.3	28.8	2.6	254	1,406	1,075	1.0	2,052	4,340	.42	2.63	1.1	6
76		1 cup	133	61	270	5	14	8.9	3.6	.3	32	176	134	.1	257	540	.05	.33	.1	1
77		3-fl oz container	50	61	100	2	5	3.4	1.4	.1	12	66	51	Trace	96	200	.02	.12	Trace	Trace
78	Soft serve (frozen custard)	1 cup	173	60	375	7	23	13.5	5.9	.6	38	236	199	.4	338	790	.08	.45	.2	1
79	Rich (about 16% fat), hardened.	1/2 gal	1,188	59	2,805	33	190	118.3	47.8	4.3	256	1,213	927	.8	1,771	7,200	.36	2.27	.9	5
80		1 cup	148	59	350	4	24	14.7	6.0	.5	32	151	115	.1	221	900	.04	.28	.1	1
	Ice milk:																			
81	Hardened (about 4.3% fat)	1/2 gal	1,048	69	1,470	41	45	28.1	11.3	1.0	232	1,409	1,035	1.5	2,117	1,710	.61	2.78	.9	6
82		1 cup	131	69	185	5	6	3.5	1.4	.1	29	176	129	.1	265	210	.08	.35	.1	1

(A)	(B)		(C)	(D)	(E)	(F)	(G)	(H)	(I)	(J)	(K)	(L)	(M)	(N)	(O)	(P)	(Q)	(R)	(S)
83	Soft serve (about 2.6% fat)	1 cup	175	70	225	8	5	2.9	1.2	0.7	38	274	202	0.3	412	180	0.12	0.54	0.2	1
84	Sherbet (about 2% fat)	1/2 gal	1,542	66	2,160	17	31	19.0	7.7		469	827	594	2.5	1,585	1,480	.26	.71	1.0	31
85		1 cup	193	66	270	2	4	2.4	1.0		59	103	74	.3	198	190	.03	.09	.1	4
	Milk desserts, other:																			
	Puddings:																			
86	Custard, baked	1 cup	265	77	305	14	15	6.8	5.4	.7	29	297	310	1.1	387	930	.11	.50	.3	1
	From home recipe:																			
	Starch base:																			
87	Chocolate	1 cup	260	66	385	8	12	7.6	3.3	.3	67	250	255	1.3	445	390	.05	.36	.3	1
88	Vanilla (blancmange)	1 cup	255	76	285	9	10	6.2	2.5	.2	41	298	232	Trace	352	410	.08	.41	.3	2
89	Tapioca cream	1 cup	165	72	220	8	8	4.1	2.5	.5	28	173	180	.7	223	480	.07	.30	.2	2
	From mix (chocolate) and milk:																			
90	Regular (cooked)	1 cup	260	70	320	9	8	4.3	2.6	.2	59	265	247	.8	354	340	.05	.39	.3	2
91	Instant	1 cup	260	69	325	8	7	3.6	2.2	.3	63	374	237	1.3	335	340	.08	.39	.3	2
	Yogurt:																			
	With added milk solids:																			
	Made with lowfat milk:																			
92	Fruit-flavored	1 container, net wt., 8 oz	227	75	230	10	3	1.8	.6	.1	42	343	269	.2	439	[10]120	.08	.40	.2	1
93	Plain	1 container, net wt., 8 oz	227	85	145	12	4	2.3	.8	.1	16	415	326	.2	531	[10]150	.10	.49	.3	2
	Made with nonfat milk:																			
94		1 container, net wt., 8 oz	227	85	125	13	Trace	.3	.1	Trace	17	452	355	.2	579	[10]120	.11	.53	.3	2
	Without added milk solids:																			
95	Made with whole milk	1 container, net wt., 8 oz	227	88	140	8	7	4.8	1.7	.1	11	274	215	.1	351	280	.07	.32	.2	1

EGGS

(A)	(B)		(C)	(D)	(E)	(F)	(G)	(H)	(I)	(J)	(K)	(L)	(M)	(N)	(O)	(P)	(Q)	(R)	(S)
	Eggs, large (24 oz per dozen):																			
	Raw:																			
96	Whole, without shell	1 egg	50	75	80	6	6	1.7	2.0	.6	1	28	90	1.0	65	260	.04	.15	Trace	0
97	White	1 white	33	88	15	3	Trace				Trace	4	4	Trace	45	0	Trace	.09	Trace	0
98	Yolk	1 yolk	17	49	65	3	6	1.7	2.1	.6	Trace	26	86	.9	15	310	.04	.07	Trace	0
	Cooked:																			
99	Fried in butter	1 egg	46	72	85	5	6	2.4	2.2	.6	1	26	80	.9	58	290	.03	.13	Trace	0
100	Hard-cooked, shell removed	1 egg	50	75	80	6	6	1.7	2.0	.6	1	28	90	.9	65	260	.04	.14	Trace	0
101	Poached	1 egg	50	74	80	6	6	1.7	2.0	.6	1	28	90	1.0	65	260	.04	.13	Trace	0
102	Scrambled (milk added) in butter. Also omelet.	1 egg	64	76	95	6	7	2.8	2.3	.6	1	47	97	.9	85	310	.04	.16	Trace	0

FATS, OILS, RELATED PRODUCTS

(A)	(B)		(C)	(D)	(E)	(F)	(G)	(H)	(I)	(J)	(K)	(L)	(M)	(N)	(O)	(P)	(Q)	(R)	(S)
	Butter:																			
	Regular (1 brick or 4 sticks per lb):																			
103	Stick (1/2 cup)	1 stick	113	16	815	1	92	57.3	23.1	2.1	Trace	27	26	.2	29	[11]3,470	.01	.04	Trace	0
104	Tablespoon (about 1/8 stick)	1 tbsp	14	16	100	Trace	12	7.2	2.9	.3	Trace	3	3	Trace	4	[11]430	Trace	Trace	Trace	0
105	Pat (1 in square, 1/3 in high; 90 per lb)	1 pat	5	16	35	Trace	4	2.5	1.0	.1	Trace	1	1	Trace	1	[11]150	Trace	Trace	Trace	0
	Whipped (6 sticks or two 8-oz containers per lb):																			
106	Stick (1/2 cup)	1 stick	76	16	540	1	61	38.2	15.4	1.4	Trace	18	17	.1	20	[11]2,310	Trace	.03	Trace	0
107	Tablespoon (about 1/8 stick)	1 tbsp	9	16	65	Trace	8	4.7	1.9	.2	Trace	2	2	Trace	2	[11]290	Trace	Trace	Trace	0
108	Pat (1 1/4 in square, 1/3 in high; 120 per lb)	1 pat	4	16	25	Trace	3	1.9	.8	.1	Trace	1	1	Trace	1	[11]120	0	Trace	Trace	0

[3]Applies to product without vitamin A added.
[4]Applies to product with added vitamin A. Without added vitamin A, value is 20 International Units (I.U.).
[5]Yields 1 qt of fluid milk when reconstituted according to package directions.
[6]Applies to product with added vitamin A.
[7]Weight applies to product with label claim of 1 1/3 cups equal 3.2 oz.
[8]Applies to products made from thick shake mixes and that do not contain added ice cream. Products made from milk shake mixes are higher in fat and usually contain added ice cream.
[9]Content of fat, vitamin A, and carbohydrate varies. Consult the label when precise values are needed for special diets.
[10]Applies to product made with milk containing no added vitamin A.
[11]Applies to product made with milk containing added vitamin A.
[11]Based on year-round average.

189

FATS, OILS; RELATED PRODUCTS—Con.

(A)	(B)	Grams	(C) Per cent	(D) Calories	(E) Grams	(F) Grams	(G) Grams	(H) Grams	(I) Grams	(J) Grams	(K) Milligrams	(L) Milligrams	(M) Milligrams	(N) Milligrams	(O) International units	(P) Milligrams	(Q) Milligrams	(R) Milligrams	(S) Milligrams
109	Fats, cooking (vegetable shortenings). 1 cup	200	0	1,770	0	200	48.8	88.2	48.4	0	0	0	0	0	—	0	0	0	0
110	1 tbsp	13	0	110	0	13	3.2	5.7	3.1	0	0	0	0	0	—	0	0	0	0
111	Lard. 1 cup	205	0	1,850	0	205	81.0	83.8	20.5	0	0	0	0	0	0	0	0	0	0
112	1 tbsp	13	0	115	0	13	5.1	5.3	1.3	0	0	0	0	0	0	0	0	0	0
	Margarine:																		
	Regular (1 brick or 4 sticks per lb):																		
113	Stick (1/2 cup)	113	16	815	1	92	16.7	42.9	24.9	Trace	27	26	.2	29	[12]3,750	.01	.04	Trace	0
114	Tablespoon (about 1/8 stick)	14	16	100	Trace	12	2.1	5.3	3.1	Trace	3	3	Trace	4	[12]470	Trace	Trace	Trace	0
115	Pat (1 in square, 1/3 in high; 90 per lb)	5	16	35	Trace	4	.7	1.9	1.1	Trace	1	1	Trace	1	[12]170	Trace	Trace	Trace	0
116	Soft, two 8-oz containers per lb. 1 container	227	16	1,635	1	184	32.5	71.5	65.4	1	53	52	.4	59	[12]7,500	.01	.08	.1	0
117	1 tbsp	14	16	100	Trace	12	2.0	4.5	4.1	Trace	3	3	Trace	4	[12]470	Trace	Trace	Trace	0
	Whipped (6 sticks per lb):																		
118	Stick (1/2 cup)	76	16	545	Trace	61	11.2	28.7	16.7	Trace	18	17	.1	20	[12]2,500	Trace	.03	Trace	0
119	Tablespoon (about 1/8 stick)	9	16	70	Trace	8	1.4	3.6	2.1	Trace	2	2	Trace	2	[12]310	Trace	Trace	Trace	0
	Oils, salad or cooking:																		
120	Corn. 1 cup	218	0	1,925	0	218	27.7	53.6	125.1	0	0	0	0	0	—	0	0	0	0
121	1 tbsp	14	0	120	0	14	1.7	3.3	7.8	0	0	0	0	0	—	0	0	0	0
122	Olive. 1 cup	216	0	1,910	0	216	30.7	154.4	17.7	0	0	0	0	0	—	0	0	0	0
123	1 tbsp	14	0	120	0	14	1.9	9.7	1.1	0	0	0	0	0	—	0	0	0	0
124	Peanut. 1 cup	216	0	1,910	0	216	37.4	98.5	67.0	0	0	0	0	0	—	0	0	0	0
125	1 tbsp	14	0	120	0	14	2.3	6.2	4.2	0	0	0	0	0	—	0	0	0	0
126	Safflower. 1 cup	218	0	1,925	0	218	20.5	25.9	159.8	0	0	0	0	0	—	0	0	0	0
127	1 tbsp	14	0	120	0	14	1.3	1.6	10.0	0	0	0	0	0	—	0	0	0	0
128	Soybean oil, hydrogenated (partially hardened). 1 cup	218	0	1,925	0	218	31.8	93.1	75.6	0	0	0	0	0	—	0	0	0	0
129	1 tbsp	14	0	120	0	14	2.0	5.8	4.7	0	0	0	0	0	—	0	0	0	0
130	Soybean-cottonseed oil blend, hydrogenated. 1 cup	218	0	1,925	0	218	38.2	63.0	99.6	0	0	0	0	0	—	0	0	0	0
131	1 tbsp	14	0	120	0	14	2.4	3.9	6.2	0	0	0	0	0	—	0	0	0	0
	Salad dressings:																		
	Commercial:																		
	Blue cheese:																		
132	Regular. 1 tbsp	15	32	75	1	8	1.6	1.7	3.8	1	12	11	Trace	6	30	Trace	.02	Trace	Trace
133	Low calorie (5 Cal per tsp). 1 tbsp	16	84	10	Trace	1	.5	.3	Trace	Trace	10	8	Trace	5	30	Trace	.01	Trace	Trace
	French:																		
134	Regular. 1 tbsp	16	39	65	Trace	6	1.1	1.3	3.2	3	2	2	.1	13	—	—	—	—	—
135	Low calorie (5 Cal per tsp). 1 tbsp	16	77	15	Trace	1	.1	.1	.4	2	2	2	.1	13	—	—	—	—	—
	Italian:																		
136	Regular. 1 tbsp	15	28	85	Trace	9	1.6	1.9	4.7	1	2	1	Trace	2	Trace	Trace	Trace	Trace	—
137	Low calorie (2 Cal per tsp). 1 tbsp	15	90	10	Trace	1	.1	.1	.4	Trace	Trace	1	Trace	2	Trace	Trace	Trace	Trace	—
138	Mayonnaise. 1 tbsp	14	15	100	Trace	11	2.0	2.4	5.6	Trace	3	4	.1	5	40	Trace	.01	Trace	—
	Mayonnaise type:																		
139	Regular. 1 tbsp	15	41	65	Trace	6	1.1	1.4	3.2	2	2	4	Trace	1	30	Trace	Trace	Trace	Trace
140	Low calorie (8 Cal per tsp). 1 tbsp	16	81	20	Trace	2	.4	.4	1.0	2	3	4	Trace	1	40	Trace	Trace	Trace	Trace
141	Tartar sauce, regular. 1 tbsp	14	34	75	Trace	8	1.1	1.8	4.1	1	3	4	.1	11	30	Trace	Trace	Trace	Trace
	Thousand Island:																		
142	Regular. 1 tbsp	16	32	80	Trace	8	1.4	1.7	4.0	2	2	3	.1	18	50	Trace	Trace	Trace	Trace
143	Low calorie (10 Cal per tsp). 1 tbsp	15	68	25	Trace	2	.4	.4	1.0	2	2	3	.1	17	50	Trace	Trace	Trace	Trace
144	From home recipe: Cooked type[13]. 1 tbsp	16	68	25	1	2	.5	.6	.3	2	14	15	.1	19	80	.01	.03	Trace	Trace

FISH, SHELLFISH, MEAT, POULTRY: RELATED PRODUCTS

(A)	(B)	Grams	(C)	(D)	(E)	(F)	(G)	(H)	(I)	(J)	(K)	(L)	(M)	(N)	(O)	(P)	(Q)	(R)	(S)
	Fish and shellfish:																		
145	Bluefish, baked with butter — 3 oz	85	68	135	22	4	—	—	—	0	25	244	0.6	—	40	0.09	0.08	1.6	—
	Clams:																		
146	Raw, meat only — 3 oz	85	82	65	11	1	—	—	—	2	59	138	5.2	154	90	.08	.15	1.1	8
147	Canned, solids and liquid — 3 oz	85	86	45	7	1	—	—	—	2	47	116	3.5	119	—	.01	.09	.9	—
148	Crabmeat (white or king), canned, not pressed down — 1 cup	135	77	135	24	3	—	—	—	1	61	246	1.1	149	—	.11	.11	2.6	—
149	Fish sticks, breaded, cooked, frozen (stick, 4 by 1 by 1/2 in) — 1 fish stick or 1 oz	28	66	50	5	3	—	—	—	2	3	47	.1	—	0	.01	.02	.5	—
150	Haddock, breaded, fried[13] — 1 fillet	85	66	140	17	5	1.4	2.2	1.2	5	34	210	1.0	296	—	.03	.06	2.7	2
151	Ocean perch, breaded, fried[13] — 1 fillet	85	59	195	16	11	2.7	4.4	2.3	6	28	192	1.1	242	—	.10	.10	1.6	—
152	Oysters, raw, meat only (13-19 medium Selects) — 1 cup	240	85	160	20	4	1.3	.2	.1	8	226	343	13.2	290	740	.34	.43	6.0	—
153	Salmon, pink, canned, solids and liquid — 3 oz	85	71	120	17	5	.9	.8	.1	0	[14]167	243	.7	307	60	.03	.16	6.8	—
154	Sardines, Atlantic, canned in oil, drained solids — 3 oz	85	62	175	20	9	3.0	2.5	.5	0	[14]372	424	2.5	502	190	.02	.17	4.6	—
155	Scallops, frozen, breaded, fried, reheated[15] — 6 scallops	90	60	175	16	8	—	—	—	9	—	—	—	—	—	—	—	—	—
156	Shad, baked with butter or margarine, bacon — 3 oz	85	64	170	20	10	—	—	—	0	20	266	.5	320	30	.11	.22	7.3	—
	Shrimp:																		
157	Canned meat — 3 oz	85	70	100	21	1	.1	.1	Trace	1	98	224	2.6	104	50	.01	.03	1.5	—
158	French fried[15] — 3 oz	85	57	190	17	9	2.3	3.7	2.0	9	61	162	1.7	195	—	.03	.07	2.3	—
159	Tuna, canned in oil, drained solids — 3 oz	85	61	170	24	7	1.7	1.7	.7	0	7	199	1.6	—	70	.04	.10	10.1	—
160	Tuna salad[16] — 1 cup	205	70	350	30	22	4.3	6.3	6.7	7	41	291	2.7	—	590	.08	.23	10.3	2
	Meat and meat products:																		
161	Bacon, (20 slices per lb, raw), broiled or fried, crisp — 2 slices	15	8	85	4	8	2.5	3.7	.7	Trace	2	34	.5	35	0	.08	.05	.8	—
	Beef, cooked: Cuts braised, simmered or pot roasted:																		
162	Lean and fat (piece, 2 1/2 by 2 1/2 by 3/4 in) — 3 oz	85	53	245	23	16	6.8	6.5	.4	0	10	114	2.9	184	30	.04	.18	3.6	—
163	Lean only from item 162 — 2.5 oz	72	62	140	22	5	2.1	1.8	.2	0	10	108	2.7	176	10	.04	.17	3.3	—
	Ground beef, broiled:																		
164	Lean with 10% fat — 3 oz or patty 3 by 5/8 in	85	60	185	23	10	4.0	3.9	.3	0	10	196	3.0	261	20	.08	.20	5.1	—
165	Lean with 21% fat — 2.9 oz or patty 3 by 5/8 in	82	54	235	20	17	7.0	6.7	.4	0	9	159	2.6	221	30	.07	.17	4.4	—
	Roast, oven cooked, no liquid: Relatively fat, such as rib:																		
166	Lean and fat (2 pieces, 4 1/8 by 2 1/4 by 1/4 in) — 3 oz	85	40	375	17	33	14.0	13.6	.8	0	8	158	2.2	189	70	.05	.13	3.1	—
167	Lean only from item 166 — 1.8 oz	51	57	125	14	7	3.0	2.5	.3	0	6	131	1.8	161	10	.04	.11	2.6	—
	Relatively lean, such as heel of round:																		
168	Lean and fat (2 pieces, 4 1/8 by 2 1/4 by 1/4 in) — 3 oz	85	62	165	25	7	2.8	2.7	.2	0	11	208	3.2	279	10	.06	.19	4.5	—

[11] Based on average vitamin A content of fortified margarine. Federal specifications for fortified margarine require a minimum of 15,000 International Units (I.U.) of vitamin A per pound.
[12] Fatty acid values apply to product made with regular-type margarine.
[13] Dipped in egg, milk or water, and breadcrumbs; fried in vegetable shortening.
[14] If bones are discarded, value for calcium will be greatly reduced.
[15] Dipped in egg, breadcrumbs, and flour or batter.
[16] Prepared with tuna, celery, salad dressing (mayonnaise type), pickle, onion, and egg.
[17] Outer layer of fat on the cut was removed to within approximately 1/2 in of the lean. Deposits of fat within the cut were not removed.

(A)	(B)	Grams	(C) Per cent	(D) Cal-ories	(E) Grams	(F) Grams	(G) Grams	(H) Grams	(I) Grams	(J) Grams	(K) Milli-grams	(L) Milli-grams	(M) Milli-grams	(N) Milli-grams	(O) Inter-national units	(P) Milli-grams	(Q) Milli-grams	(R) Milli-grams	(S) Milli-grams
	FISH, SHELLFISH, MEAT, POULTRY: RELATED PRODUCTS—Con.																		
	Meat and meat products—Continued																		
	Beef," cooked—Continued																		
	Roast, oven cooked, no liquid added—Continued																		
	Relatively lean such as heel of round—Continued																		
169	Lean only from item 168--- 2.8 oz	78	65	125	24	3	1.2	1.0	0.1	0	10	199	3.0	268	Trace	0.06	0.18	4.3	—
	Steak:																		
	Relatively fat—sirloin, broiled:																		
170	Lean and fat (piece, 2 1/2 by 2 1/2 by 3/4 in)--- 3 oz	85	44	330	20	27	11.3	11.1	.6	0	9	162	2.5	220	50	.05	.15	4.0	—
171	Lean only from item 170--- 2.0 oz	56	59	115	18	4	1.8	1.6	.2	0	7	146	2.2	202	10	.05	.14	3.6	—
	Relatively lean—round, braised:																		
172	Lean and fat (piece, 4 1/8 by 2 1/4 by 1/2 in)--- 3 oz	85	55	220	24	13	5.5	5.2	.4	0	10	213	3.0	272	20	.07	.19	4.8	—
173	Lean only from item 172--- 2.4 oz	68	61	130	21	4	1.7	1.5	.2	0	9	182	2.5	238	10	.05	.16	4.1	—
	Beef, canned:																		
174	Corned beef--- 3 oz	85	59	185	22	10	4.9	4.5	.1	0	17	90	3.7	—	—	.01	.20	2.9	—
175	Corned beef hash--- 1 cup	220	67	400	19	25	11.9	10.9	.5	24	29	147	4.4	440	—	.02	.20	4.6	—
176	Beef, dried, chipped--- 2 1/2-oz jar	71	48	145	24	4	2.1	2.0	.1	0	14	287	3.6	142	—	.05	.23	2.7	0
177	Beef and vegetable stew--- 1 cup	245	82	220	16	11	4.9	4.5	.2	15	29	184	2.9	613	2,400	.15	.17	4.7	17
178	Beef potpie (home recipe), baked (piece, 1/3 of 9-in diam. pie)--- 1 piece	210	55	515	21	30	7.9	12.8	6.7	39	29	149	3.8	334	1,720	.30	.30	5.5	6
179	Chili con carne with beans, canned--- 1 cup	255	72	340	19	16	7.5	6.8	.3	31	82	321	4.3	594	150	.08	.18	3.3	—
180	Chop suey with beef and pork (home recipe)--- 1 cup	250	75	300	26	17	8.5	6.2	.7	13	60	248	4.8	425	600	.28	.38	5.0	33
181	Heart, beef, lean, braised--- 3 oz	85	61	160	27	5	1.5	1.1	.6	1	5	154	5.0	197	20	.21	1.04	6.5	1
	Lamb, cooked:																		
	Chop, rib (cut 3 per lb with bone), broiled:																		
182	Lean and fat--- 3.1 oz	89	43	360	18	32	14.8	12.1	1.2	0	8	139	1.0	200	—	.11	.19	4.1	—
183	Lean only from item 182--- 2 oz	57	60	120	16	6	2.5	2.1	.2	0	6	121	1.1	174	—	.09	.15	3.4	—
	Leg, roasted:																		
184	Lean and fat (2 pieces, 4 1/8 by 2 1/4 by 1/4 in).--- 3 oz	85	54	235	22	16	7.3	6.0	.6	0	9	177	1.4	241	—	.13	.23	4.7	—
185	Lean only from item 184--- 2.5 oz	71	62	130	20	5	2.1	1.8	.2	0	9	169	1.4	227	—	.12	.21	4.4	—
	Shoulder, roasted:																		
186	Lean and fat (3 pieces, 2 1/2 by 2 1/2 by 1/4 in)--- 3 oz	85	50	285	18	23	10.8	8.8	.9	0	9	146	1.0	206	—	.11	.20	4.0	—
187	Lean only from item 186--- 2.3 oz	64	61	130	17	6	3.6	2.3	.2	0	8	140	1.0	193	—	.10	.18	3.7	—
188	Liver, beef, fried[5] (slice, 6 1/2 by 2 3/8 by 3/8 in)--- 3 oz	85	56	195	22	9	2.5	3.5	.9	5	9	405	7.5	323	[2]45,390	.22	3.56	14.0	23
	Pork, cured, cooked:																		
189	Ham, light cure, lean and fat, roasted (2 pieces, 4 1/8 by 2 1/4 by 1/4 in).[2]--- 3 oz	85	54	245	18	19	6.8	7.9	1.7	0	8	146	2.2	199	0	.40	.15	3.1	—
	Luncheon meat:																		
190	Boiled ham, slice (8 per 8-oz pkg.).--- 1 oz	28	59	65	5	5	1.7	2.0	.4	0	3	47	.8	—	0	.12	.04	.7	—
191	Canned, spiced or unspiced: Slice, approx. 3 by 2 by 1/2 in.--- 1 slice	60	55	175	9	15	5.4	6.7	1.0	1	5	65	1.3	133	0	.19	.13	1.8	—

Pork, fresh,[18] cooked:

(A)	(B) Foods, approximate measure, units, and weight	Grams	(C) Water (pct)	(D) Food energy (cal)	(E) Protein (g)	(F) Fat (g)	(G) Saturated (g)	(H) Oleic (g)	(I) Linoleic (g)	(J) Carbohydrate (g)	(K) Calcium (mg)	(L) Phosphorus (mg)	(M) Iron (mg)	(N) Potassium (mg)	(O) Vitamin A (IU)	(P) Thiamin (mg)	(Q) Riboflavin (mg)	(R) Niacin (mg)	(S) Ascorbic acid (mg)
	Chop, loin (cut 3 per lb with bone), broiled:																		
192	Lean and fat — 2.7 oz	78	42	305	19	25	8.9	10.4	2.2	0	9	209	2.7	216	0	0.75	0.22	4.5	—
193	Lean only from item 192 — 2 oz	56	53	150	17	9	3.1	3.6	.8	0	7	181	2.2	192	0	.63	.18	3.8	—
	Roast, oven cooked, no liquid added:																		
194	Lean and fat (piece, 2 1/2 by 2 1/2 by 3/4 in.) — 3 oz	85	46	310	21	24	8.7	10.2	2.2	0	9	218	2.7	233	0	.78	.22	4.8	—
195	Lean only from item 194 — 2.4 oz	68	55	175	20	10	3.5	4.1	.8	0	9	211	2.6	224	0	.73	.21	4.4	—
	Shoulder cut, simmered:																		
196	Lean and fat (3 pieces, 2 1/2 by 2 1/2 by 1/4 in.) — 3 oz	85	46	320	20	26	9.3	10.9	2.3	0	9	118	2.6	158	0	.46	.21	4.1	—
197	Lean only from item 196 — 2.2 oz	63	60	135	18	6	2.2	2.6	.6	0	8	111	2.3	146	0	.42	.19	3.7	—
	Sausages (see also Luncheon meat (items 190-191)):																		
198	Bologna, slice (8 per 8-oz pkg.) — 1 slice	28	56	85	3	8	3.0	3.4	.5	Trace	2	36	.5	65	—	.05	.06	.7	—
199	Braunschweiger, slice (6 per 6-oz pkg.) — 1 slice	28	53	90	4	8	2.6	3.4	.8	1	3	69	1.7	—	1,850	.05	.41	2.3	—
200	Brown and serve (10-11 per 8-oz pkg.), browned — 1 link	17	40	70	3	6	2.3	2.8	.7	Trace	—	—	—	—	0	—	—	—	—
201	Deviled ham, canned — 1 tbsp	13	51	45	2	4	1.5	1.8	.4	0	1	12	.3	—	0	.02	.01	.2	—
202	Frankfurter (8 per 1-lb pkg.), cooked (reheated) — 1 frankfurter	56	57	170	7	15	5.6	6.5	1.2	1	3	57	.8	—	—	.08	.11	1.4	—
203	Meat, potted (beef, chicken, turkey), canned — 1 tbsp	13	61	30	2	2	—	—	—	0	—	—	—	—	0	Trace	.03	.2	—
204	Pork link (16 per 1-lb pkg.), cooked — 1 link	13	35	60	2	6	2.1	2.4	.5	Trace	1	21	.3	35	—	.10	.04	.5	—
	Salami:																		
205	Dry type, slice (12 per 4-oz pkg.) — 1 slice	10	30	45	2	4	1.6	1.6	.1	Trace	1	28	.4	—	—	.04	.03	.5	—
206	Cooked type, slice (8 per 8-oz pkg.) — 1 slice	28	51	90	5	7	3.1	3.0	.2	Trace	3	57	.7	—	—	.07	.07	1.2	—
207	Vienna sausage (7 per 4-oz can) — 1 sausage	16	53	40	2	3	1.2	1.4	.2	Trace	1	24	.3	—	—	.01	.02	.4	—
	Veal, medium fat, cooked, bone removed:																		
208	Cutlet (4 1/8 by 2 1/4 by 1/2 in.), braised or broiled — 3 oz	85	60	185	23	9	4.0	3.4	.4	0	9	196	2.7	258	—	.06	.21	4.6	—
209	Rib (2 pieces, 4 1/8 by 2 1/4 by 1/4 in.), roasted — 3 oz	85	55	230	23	14	6.1	5.1	.6	0	10	211	2.9	259	—	.11	.26	6.6	—
	Poultry and poultry products: Chicken, cooked:																		
210	Breast, fried,[21] bones removed, 1/2 breast (3.3 oz with bones) — 2.8 oz	79	58	160	26	5	1.4	1.8	1.1	1	9	218	1.3	—	70	.04	.17	11.6	—
211	Drumstick, fried,[21] bones removed (2 oz with bones) — 1.3 oz	38	55	90	12	4	1.1	1.3	.9	Trace	6	89	.9	—	50	.03	.15	2.7	—
212	Half broiler, broiled, bones removed (10.4 oz with bones) — 6.2 oz	176	71	240	42	7	2.2	2.5	1.3	0	16	355	3.0	483	160	.09	.34	15.5	—
213	Chicken, canned, boneless — 3 oz	85	65	170	18	10	3.2	3.8	2.0	0	18	210	1.3	117	200	.03	.11	3.7	3
214	Chicken a la king, cooked (home recipe) — 1 cup	245	68	470	27	34	12.7	14.3	3.3	12	127	358	2.5	404	1,130	.10	.42	5.4	12
215	Chicken and noodles, cooked (home recipe) — 1 cup	240	71	365	22	18	5.9	7.1	3.5	26	26	247	2.2	149	430	.05	.17	4.3	Trace

[17]Outer layer of fat on the cut was removed to within approximately 1/2 in. of the lean. Deposits of fat within the cut were not removed.
[18]Crust made with vegetable shortening and enriched flour.
[19]Regular-type margarine used.
[20]Value varies widely.
[21]About one-fourth of the outer layer of fat on the cut was removed. Deposits of fat within the cut were not removed.
[22]Vegetable shortening used.

FISH, SHELLFISH, MEAT, POULTRY, RELATED PRODUCTS—Con.

(A)	(B)	Grams	(C) Per-cent	(D) Cal-ories	(E) Grams	(F) Grams	(G) Grams	(H) Grams	(I) Grams	(J) Grams	(K) Milli-grams	(L) Milli-grams	(M) Milli-grams	(N) Milli-grams	(O) Inter-national units	(P) Milli-grams	(Q) Milli-grams	(R) Milli-grams	(S) Milli-grams
	Poultry and poultry products—Continued																		
	Chicken chow mein:																		
216	Canned——————— 1 cup———	250	89	95	7	Trace	2.4	3.4		18	45	35	1.3	418	150	0.05	0.10	1.0	13
217	From home recipe——— 1 cup———	250	78	255	31	10				10	58	293	2.5	473	280	.08	.23	4.3	10
218	Chicken potpie (home recipe), baked, 1¼ piece (1/3 or 9-in diam. pie)——— 1 piece———	232	57	545	23	31	11.3	10.9	5.6	42	70	232	3.0	343	3,090	.34	.31	5.5	5
	Turkey, roasted, flesh without skin:																		
219	Dark meat, piece, 2 1/2 by 1 5/8 by 1/4 in.——— 4 pieces———	85	61	175	26	7	2.1	1.5	1.5	0			2.0	338		.03	.20	3.6	—
220	Light meat, piece, 4 by 2 by 1/4 in.——— 2 pieces———	85	62	150	28	3	.9	.6	.7	0			1.0	349		.04	.12	9.4	—
	Light and dark meat:																		
221	Chopped or diced——— 1 cup———	140	61	265	44	9	2.5	1.7	1.8	0		11	351	2.5	514		.07	.25	10.8	—
222	Pieces (1 slice white meat, 4 by 2 by 1/4 in with 2 slices dark meat, 2 1/2 by 1 5/8 by 1/4 in).——— 3 pieces———	85	61	160	27	5	1.5	1.0	1.1	0	7	213	1.5	312		.04	.15	6.5	—

FRUITS AND FRUIT PRODUCTS

(A)	(B)	Grams	(C) Per-cent	(D) Cal-ories	(E) Grams	(F) Grams	(G) Grams	(H) Grams	(I) Grams	(J) Grams	(K) Milli-grams	(L) Milli-grams	(M) Milli-grams	(N) Milli-grams	(O) Inter-national units	(P) Milli-grams	(Q) Milli-grams	(R) Milli-grams	(S) Milli-grams
	Apples, raw, unpeeled, without cores:																		
223	2 3/4-in diam. (about 3 per lb with cores)——— 1 apple———	138	84	80	Trace	1	—	—	—	20	10	14	.4	152	120	.04	.03	.1	6
224	3 1/4-in diam. (about 2 per lb with cores)——— 1 apple———	212	84	125	Trace	1	—	—	—	31	15	21	.6	233	190	.06	.04	.2	8
225	Applejuice, bottled or canned²——— 1 cup———	248	88	120	Trace	Trace	—	—	—	30	15	22	1.5	250	—	.02	.05	.2	2[52]
	Applesauce, canned:																		
226	Sweetened——— 1 cup———	255	76	230	1	Trace	—	—	—	61	10	13	1.3	166	100	.05	.03	.1	2[13]
227	Unsweetened——— 1 cup———	244	89	100	Trace	Trace	—	—	—	26	10	12	1.2	190	100	.05	.02	.1	2[13]
	Apricots:																		
228	Raw, without pits (about 12 per lb with pits)——— 3 apricots———	107	85	55	1	Trace	—	—	—	14	18	25	.5	301	2,890	.03	.04	.6	11
229	Canned in heavy sirup (halves and sirup).——— 1 cup———	258	77	220	2	Trace	—	—	—	57	28	39	.8	604	4,490	.05	.05	1.0	10
	Dried:																		
230	Uncooked (28 large or 37 medium halves per cup).——— 1 cup———	130	25	340	7	1	—	—	—	86	87	140	7.2	1,273	14,170	.01	.21	4.3	16
231	Cooked, unsweetened, fruit and liquid.——— 1 cup———	250	76	215	4	1	—	—	—	54	55	88	4.5	795	7,500	.01	.13	2.5	8
232	Apricot nectar, canned——— 1 cup———	251	85	145	1	Trace	—	—	—	37	23	30	.5	379	2,380	.03	.03	.5	2[36]
	Avocados, raw, whole, without skins and seeds:																		
233	California, mid- and late-winter (with skin and seed, 3 1/8-in diam.; wt. 10 oz).——— 1 avocado———	216	74	370	5	37	5.5	22.0	3.7	13	22	91	1.3	1,303	630	.24	.43	3.5	30
234	Florida, late summer and fall (with skin and seed, 3 5/8-in diam.; wt. 1 lb).——— 1 avocado———	304	78	390	4	33	6.7	15.7	5.3	27	30	128	1.8	1,836	880	.33	.61	4.9	43
235	Banana without peel (about 2.6 per lb with peel).——— 1 banana———	119	76	100	1	Trace	—	—	—	26	10	31	.8	440	230	.06	.07	.8	12
236	Banana flakes——— 1 tbsp———	6	3	20	Trace	Trace	—	—	—	5	2	6	.2	92	50	.01	.01	.2	Trace

(A)	(B)	(C)	(D)	(E)	(F)	(G)	(H)	(I)	(J)	(K)	(L)	(M)	(N)	(O)	(P)	(Q)	(R)	(S)
237	Blackberries, raw -- 1 cup	144	85	85	2	1	—	—	—	19	46	27	1.3	245	290	0.04	0.06	0.6	30
238	Blueberries, raw -- 1 cup	145	83	90	1	1	—	—	—	22	22	19	1.5	117	150	.04	.09	.7	20
	Cantaloup. See Muskmelons (item 271).																		
	Cherries:																		
239	Sour (tart), red, pitted, canned, water pack -- 1 cup	244	88	105	2	Trace	—	—	—	26	37	32	.7	317	1,660	.07	.05	.5	12
240	Sweet, raw, without pits and stems -- 10 cherries	68	80	45	1	Trace	—	—	—	12	15	13	.3	129	70	.03	.04	.3	7
241	Cranberry juice cocktail, bottled, sweetened -- 1 cup	253	83	165	Trace	Trace	—	—	—	42	13	8	.8	25	Trace	.03	.03	.1	[27]81
242	Cranberry sauce, sweetened, canned, strained -- 1 cup	277	62	405	Trace	1	—	—	—	104	17	11	.6	83	60	.03	.03	.1	6
	Dates:																		
243	Whole, without pits -- 10 dates	80	23	220	2	Trace	—	—	—	58	47	50	2.4	518	40	.07	.08	1.8	0
244	Chopped -- 1 cup	178	23	490	4	1	—	—	—	130	105	112	5.3	1,153	90	.16	.18	3.9	0
245	Fruit cocktail, canned, in heavy syrup -- 1 cup	255	80	195	1	Trace	—	—	—	50	23	31	1.0	411	360	.05	.03	1.0	5
	Grapefruit:																		
	Raw, medium, 3 3/4-in diam. (about 1 lb 1 oz):																		
246	Pink or red[18] -- 1/2 grapefruit with peel[18]	241	89	50	1	Trace	—	—	—	13	20	20	.5	166	540	.05	.02	.2	44
247	White[18] -- 1/2 grapefruit with peel[18]	241	89	45	1	Trace	—	—	—	12	19	19	.5	159	10	.05	.02	.2	44
248	Canned, sections with sirup -- 1 cup	254	81	180	2	Trace	—	—	—	45	33	36	.8	343	30	.08	.05	.5	76
249	Grapefruit juice: Raw, pink, red, or white -- 1 cup	246	90	95	1	Trace	—	—	—	23	22	37	.5	399	(20)	.10	.05	.5	93
	Canned, white:																		
250	Unsweetened -- 1 cup	247	89	100	1	Trace	—	—	—	24	20	35	1.0	400	20	.07	.05	.5	84
251	Sweetened -- 1 cup	250	86	135	1	Trace	—	—	—	32	20	35	1.0	405	30	.08	.05	.5	78
	Frozen concentrate, unsweetened:																		
252	Undiluted, 6-fl oz can -- 1 can	207	62	300	4	1	—	—	—	72	70	124	.8	1,250	60	.29	.12	1.4	286
253	Diluted with 3 parts water by volume -- 1 can	247	89	100	1	1	—	—	—	24	25	42	.2	420	20	.10	.04	.5	96
254	Dehydrated crystals, prepared with water (1 lb yields about 1 gal) -- 1 cup	247	90	100	1	Trace	—	—	—	24	22	40	.2	412	20	.10	.05	.5	91
	Grapes, European type (adherent skin), raw:																		
255	Thompson Seedless -- 10 grapes	50	81	35	Trace	Trace	—	—	—	9	6	10	.2	87	50	.03	.02	.2	2
256	Tokay and Emperor, seeded types -- 10 grapes[19]	60	81	40	Trace	Trace	—	—	—	10	7	11	.2	99	60	.03	.02	.2	2
	Grapejuice:																		
257	Canned or bottled -- 1 cup	253	83	165	1	Trace	—	—	—	42	28	30	.8	293	—	.10	.05	.5	[23]Trace
	Frozen concentrate, sweetened:																		
258	Undiluted, 6-fl oz can -- 1 can	216	53	395	1	Trace	—	—	—	100	22	32	.9	255	40	.13	.22	1.5	[1]132
259	Diluted with 3 parts water by volume -- 1 can	250	86	135	1	Trace	—	—	—	33	8	10	.3	85	10	.05	.08	.5	[1]10
260	Grape drink, canned -- 1 cup	250	86	135	Trace	Trace	—	—	—	35	8	10	.3	88	10	[32].03	[32].03	.3	(32)
261	Lemon, raw, size 165, without peel and seeds (about 4 per lb with peels and seeds) -- 1 lemon	74	90	20	1	Trace	—	—	—	6	19	12	.4	102	10	.03	.01	.1	39
	Lemon juice:																		
262	Raw -- 1 cup	244	91	60	1	Trace	—	—	—	20	17	24	.5	344	50	.07	.02	.2	112
263	Canned or bottled, unsweetened -- 1 cup	244	92	55	1	Trace	—	—	—	19	17	24	.5	344	50	.07	.02	.2	102
264	Frozen, single strength, unsweetened, 6-fl oz can -- 1 can	183	92	40	1	Trace	—	—	—	13	13	16	.5	258	40	.05	.02	.2	81
	Lemonade concentrate, frozen:																		
265	Undiluted, 6-fl oz can -- 1 can	219	49	425	Trace	Trace	—	—	—	112	9	13	.4	153	40	.05	.06	.7	66
266	Diluted with 4 1/3 parts water by volume -- 1 cup	248	89	105	Trace	Trace	—	—	—	28	2	3	.1	40	10	.01	.02	.2	17

[18]Crust made with vegetable shortening and enriched flour.
[21]Also applies to pasteurized apple cider.
[23]Applies to product without added ascorbic acid. For value of product with added ascorbic acid, refer to label.
[26]Based on product without added ascorbic acid.
[27]Based on product with label claim of 45% of U.S. RDA in 6 fl oz.
[28]Based on product with label claim of 100% of U.S. RDA in 6 fl oz.
[29]Weight includes peel and membranes between sections. Without these parts, the weight of the edible portion is 123 g for item 246 and 118 g for item 247.
[30]For white-fleshed varieties, value is about 20 International Units (I.U.) per cup; for red-fleshed varieties, 1,080 I.U.
[31]Weight includes seeds. Without seeds, weight of the edible portion is 57 g.
[32]Applies to product without added ascorbic acid. With added ascorbic acid, based on claim that 6 fl oz of reconstituted juice contain 45% or 50% of the U.S. RDA, value in milligrams is 108 or 120 for a 6-fl oz can (item 258), 36 or 40 for 1 cup of diluted juice (item 259). For products with added thiamin and riboflavin but without added ascorbic acid, values in milligrams would be 0.60 for thiamin, 0.80 for riboflavin, and trace for ascorbic acid. For products with only ascorbic acid added, value varies with the brand. Consult the label.

(A)	(B) FRUITS AND FRUIT PRODUCTS—Con.	Grams	(C) Per-cent	(D) Cal-ories	(E) Grams	(F) Grams	(G) Grams	(H) Grams	(I) Grams	(I) Grams	(K) Milli-grams	(L) Milli-grams	(M) Milli-grams	(N) Milli-grams	(O) Inter-national units	(P) Milli-grams	(Q) Milli-grams	(R) Milli-grams	(S) Milli-grams
	Limeade concentrate, frozen:																		
267	Undiluted, 6-fl oz can --- 1 can	218	50	410	Trace	Trace	—	—	—	-108	11	13	0.2	129	Trace	0.02	0.02	0.2	26
268	Diluted with 4 1/3 parts water by volume --- 1 cup	247	89	100	Trace	Trace	—	—	—	27	3	3	Trace	32	Trace	Trace	Trace	Trace	6
	Lime juice:																		
269	Raw --- 1 cup	246	90	65	1	Trace	—	—	—	22	22	27	.5	256	20	.05	.02	.2	79
270	Canned, unsweetened --- 1 cup	246	90	65	1	Trace	—	—	—	22	22	27	.5	256	20	.05	.02	.2	52
	Muskmelons, raw, with rind, without seed cavity:																		
271	Cantaloup, orange-fleshed (with rind and seed cavity, 5-in diam., 2 1/3 lb) --- 1/2 melon with rind [33]	477	91	80	2	Trace	—	—	—	20	38	44	1.1	682	9,240	.11	.08	1.6	90
272	Honeydew (with rind and seed cavity, 6 1/2-in diam., 5 1/4 lb) --- 1/10 melon with rind [33]	226	91	50	1	Trace	—	—	—	11	21	24	.6	374	60	.06	.04	.9	34
	Oranges, all commercial varieties:																		
273	Whole, 2 5/8-in diam., without peel and seeds (about 2 1/2 per lb with peel and seeds) --- 1 orange	131	86	65	1	Trace	—	—	—	16	54	26	.5	263	260	.13	.05	.5	66
274	Sections without membranes --- 1 cup	180	86	90	2	Trace	—	—	—	22	74	36	.7	360	360	.18	.07	.7	90
	Orange juice:																		
275	Raw, all varieties --- 1 cup	248	88	110	2	Trace	—	—	—	26	27	42	.5	496	500	.22	.07	1.0	124
276	Canned, unsweetened --- 1 cup	249	87	120	2	Trace	—	—	—	28	25	45	1.0	496	500	.17	.05	.7	100
	Frozen concentrate:																		
277	Undiluted, 6-fl oz can --- 1 can	213	55	360	5	Trace	—	—	—	87	75	126	.9	1,500	1,620	.68	.11	2.8	360
278	Diluted with 3 parts water by volume --- 1 cup	249	87	120	2	Trace	—	—	—	29	25	42	.2	503	540	.23	.03	.9	120
279	Dehydrated crystals, prepared with water (1 lb yields about 1 gal) --- 1 cup	248	88	115	1	Trace	—	—	—	27	25	40	.5	518	500	.20	.07	1.0	109
	Orange and grapefruit juice: Frozen concentrate:																		
280	Undiluted, 6-fl oz can --- 1 can	210	59	330	4	1	—	—	—	78	61	99	.8	1,308	800	.48	.06	2.3	302
281	Diluted with 3 parts water by volume --- 1 cup	248	88	110	1	Trace	—	—	—	26	20	32	.2	439	270	.15	.02	.7	102
282	Papayas, raw, 1/2-in cubes --- 1 cup	140	89	55	1	Trace	—	—	—	14	28	22	.4	328	2,450	.06	.06	.4	78
	Peaches: Raw:																		
283	Whole, 2 1/2-in diam., peeled, pitted (about 4 per lb with peels and pits) --- 1 peach	100	89	40	1	Trace	—	—	—	10	9	19	.5	202	[11]1,330	.02	.05	1.0	7
284	Sliced --- 1 cup	170	89	65	1	Trace	—	—	—	16	15	32	.9	343	[11]2,260	.03	.09	1.7	12
	Canned, yellow-fleshed, solids and liquid (halves or slices):																		
285	Syrup pack --- 1 cup	256	79	200	1	Trace	—	—	—	51	10	31	.8	333	1,100	.03	.05	1.5	8
286	Water pack --- 1 cup	244	91	75	1	Trace	—	—	—	20	10	32	.7	334	1,100	.02	.07	1.5	7
	Dried:																		
287	Uncooked --- 1 cup	160	25	420	5	1	—	—	—	109	77	187	9.6	1,520	6,240	.02	.30	8.5	29
288	Cooked, unsweetened, halves and juice --- 1 cup	250	77	205	3	1	—	—	—	54	38	93	4.8	743	3,050	.01	.15	3.8	5

(A)	(B)	(C)	(D)	(E)	(F)	(G)	(H)	(I)	(J)	(K)	(L)	(M)	(N)	(O)	(P)	(Q)	(R)	(S)
	Frozen, sliced, sweetened:																	
289	10-oz container------ 1 container----	284	77	250	1	Trace	—	—	64	11	37	1.4	352	1,850	0.03	0.11	2.0	[3][4]116
290	Cup------------------ 1 cup----------	250	77	220	1	Trace	—	—	57	10	33	1.3	310	1,630	.03	.10	1.8	[3][4]103
	Pears:																	
	Raw, with skin, cored:																	
291	Bartlett, 2 1/2-in diam. (about 2 1/2 per lb with cores and stems)------ 1 pear----	164	83	100	1	1	—	—	25	13	18	.5	213	30	.03	.07	.2	7
292	Bosc, 2 1/2-in diam. (about 3 per lb with cores and stems)------ 1 pear----	141	83	85	1	1	—	—	22	11	16	.4	83	30	.03	.06	.1	6
293	D'Anjou, 3-in diam. (about 2 per lb with cores and stems)------ 1 pear----	200	83	120	1	1	—	—	31	16	22	.6	260	40	.04	.08	.2	8
294	Canned, solids and liquid, sirup pack, heavy (halves or slices)------ 1 cup----	255	80	195	1	Trace	—	—	50	13	18	.5	214	10	.03	.05	.3	3
	Pineapple:																	
295	Raw, diced------ 1 cup----	155	85	80	Trace	Trace	—	—	21	26	12	.8	226	110	.14	.05	.3	26
	Canned, heavy sirup pack, solids and liquid:																	
296	Crushed, chunks, tidbits------ 1 cup----	255	80	190	1	Trace	—	—	49	28	13	.8	245	130	.20	.05	.5	18
	Slices and liquid:																	
297	Large------ 1 slice; 2 1/4 tbsp liquid.	105	80	80	Trace	Trace	—	—	20	12	5	.3	101	50	.08	.02	.2	7
298	Medium------ 1 slices; 1 1/4 tbsp liquid.	58	80	45	Trace	Trace	—	—	11	6	3	.2	56	30	.05	.01	.1	4
299	Pineapple juice, unsweetened, canned------ 1 cup----	250	86	140	1	Trace	—	—	34	38	23	.8	373	130	.13	.05	.5	[2,7]80
	Plums:																	
	Raw, without pits:																	
300	Japanese and hybrid (2 1/8-in diam., about 6 1/2 per lb with pits)------ 1 plum----	66	87	30	Trace	Trace	—	—	8	8	12	.3	112	160	.02	.02	.3	4
301	Prune-type (1 1/2-in diam., about 15 per lb with pits)------ 1 plum----	28	79	20	Trace	Trace	—	—	6	3	5	.1	48	80	.01	.01	.1	1
	Canned, heavy sirup pack (Italian prunes), with pits and liquid:																	
302	Cup[14]------ 1 cup----	272	77	215	1	Trace	—	—	56	23	26	2.3	367	3,130	.05	.05	1.0	5
303	Portion------ 3 plums; 2 3/4 tbsp liquid.[14]	140	77	110	1	Trace	—	—	29	12	13	1.2	189	1,610	.03	.03	.5	3
	Prunes, dried, "softenized," with pits:																	
304	Uncooked------ 4 extra large or 5 large prunes.[14]	49	28	110	1	Trace	—	—	29	22	34	1.7	298	690	.04	.07	.7	1
305	Cooked, unsweetened, all sizes, fruit and liquid------ 1 cup[14]----	250	66	255	2	1	—	—	67	51	79	3.8	695	1,590	.07	.15	1.5	2
306	Prune juice, canned or bottled------ 1 cup----	256	80	195	1	Trace	—	—	49	36	51	1.8	602	—	.03	.03	1.0	5
	Raisins, seedless:																	
307	Cup, not pressed down------ 1 cup----	145	18	420	4	Trace	—	—	112	90	146	5.1	1,106	30	.16	.12	.7	1
308	Packet, 1/2 oz (1 1/2 tbsp)------ 1 packet----	14	18	40	Trace	Trace	—	—	11	9	14	.5	107	Trace	.02	.01	.1	Trace
	Raspberries, red:																	
309	Raw, capped, whole------ 1 cup----	123	84	70	1	1	—	—	17	27	27	1.1	207	160	.04	.11	1.1	31
310	Frozen, sweetened, 10-oz container------ 1 container----	284	74	280	2	1	—	—	70	37	48	1.7	284	200	.06	.17	1.7	60
	Rhubarb, cooked, added sugar:																	
311	From raw------ 1 cup----	270	63	380	1	Trace	—	—	97	211	41	1.6	548	220	.05	.14	.8	16
312	From frozen, sweetened------ 1 cup----	270	63	385	1	Trace	—	—	93	211	32	1.9	475	190	.05	.11	.5	16

[2] Based on product with label claim of 100% of U.S. RDA in 6 fl oz.

[3] Weight includes rind. Without rind, the weight of the edible portion is 272 g for item 271 and 149 g for item 272.

[4] Represents yellow-fleshed varieties. For white-fleshed varieties, value is 50 International Units (I.U.) for 1 peach, 90 I.U. for 1 cup of slices.

[5] Value represents products without added ascorbic acid. For products with added ascorbic acid, value in milligrams is 116 for a 10-oz container, 103 for 1 cup, 43 g for item 304, and 213 g for item 305.

[6] Weight includes pits. After removal of the pits, the weight of the edible portion is 258 g for item 302, 133 g for item 303, 43 g for item 304, and 213 g for item 305.

(A)	(B)	Grams	(C) Per-cent	(D) Cal-ories	(E) Grams	(F) Grams	(G) Grams	(H) Grams	(I) Grams	(J) Grams	(K) Milli-grams	(L) Milli-grams	(M) Milli-grams	(N) Milli-grams	(O) Inter-national units	(P) Milli-grams	(Q) Milli-grams	(R) Milli-grams	(S) Milli-grams
	FRUITS AND FRUIT PRODUCTS—Con.																		
	Strawberries:																		
313	Raw, whole berries, capped———— 1 cup	149	90	55	1	1	—	—	—	13	31	31	1.5	244	90	0.04	0.10	0.9	88
	Frozen, sweetened:																		
314	Sliced, 10-oz container——— 1 container	284	71	310	1	1	—	—	—	79	40	48	2.0	318	90	.06	.17	1.4	151
315	Whole, 1-lb container (about 1 3/4 cups)——— 1 container	454	76	415	1	2	—	—	—	107	59	73	2.7	472	140	.09	.27	2.3	249
316	Tangerine, raw, 2 3/8-in diam., size 176, without peel (about 4 per lb with peels and seeds)——— 1 tangerine	86	87	40	1	Trace	—	—	—	10	34	15	.3	108	360	.05	.02	.1	27
317	Tangerine juice, canned, sweet-ened——— 1 cup	249	87	125	1	Trace	—	—	—	30	44	35	.5	440	1,040	.15	.05	.2	54
318	Watermelon, raw, 4 by 8 in wedge with rind and seeds (1/16 of 32 2/3-lb melon, 10 by 16 in)——— 1 wedge with rind and seeds [17]	926	93	110	2	1	—	—	—	27	30	43	2.1	426	2,510	.13	.13	.9	30
	GRAIN PRODUCTS																		
	Bagel, 3-in diam.:																		
319	Egg——— 1 bagel	55	32	165	6	2	0.5	0.9	0.8	28	9	43	1.2	41	30	.14	.10	1.2	0
320	Water——— 1 bagel	55	29	165	6	2	.2	.4	.6	30	8	41	1.2	42	0	.15	.11	1.4	0
321	Barley, pearled, light, uncooked——— 1 cup	200	11	700	16	2	.3	.2	.8	158	32	378	4.0	320	0	.24	.10	6.2	0
	Biscuits, baking powder, 2-in diam. (enriched flour, vege-table shortening):																		
322	From home recipe——— 1 biscuit	28	27	105	2	5	1.2	2.0	1.2	13	34	49	.4	33	Trace	.08	.08	.7	Trace
323	From mix——— 1 biscuit	28	29	90	2	3	.6	1.1	.7	15	65	65	.6	32	Trace	.08	.08	.8	Trace
324	Breadcrumbs (enriched): [18] Dry, grated——— 1 cup	100	7	390	13	5	1.0	1.6	1.4	73	122	141	3.6	152	Trace	.35	.35	4.8	Trace
	Breads: Soft. See white bread (items 349-350).																		
325	Boston brown bread, canned, slice, 3 1/4 by 1/2 in. [19]——— 1 slice	45	45	95	2	1	.1	.2	.2	21	41	72	.9	131	[19]0	.06	.04	.7	0
	Cracked-wheat bread (3/4 en-riched wheat flour, 1/4 cracked wheat): [18]																		
326	Loaf, 1 lb——— 1 loaf	454	35	1,195	39	10	2.2	3.0	3.9	236	399	581	9.5	608	Trace	1.52	1.13	14.4	Trace
327	Slice (18 per loaf)——— 1 slice	25	35	65	2	1	.1	.2	.2	13	22	32	.5	34	Trace	.08	.06	.8	Trace
	French or vienna bread, en-riched: [18]																		
328	Loaf, 1 lb——— 1 loaf	454	31	1,315	41	14	3.2	4.7	4.6	251	195	386	10.0	408	Trace	1.80	1.10	15.0	Trace
	Slice:																		
329	French (5 by 2 1/2 by 1 in)——— 1 slice	35	31	100	3	1	.2	.4	.4	19	15	30	.8	32	Trace	.14	.08	1.2	Trace
330	Vienna (4 3/4 by 4 by 1/2 in)——— 1 slice	25	31	75	2	1	.2	.3	.3	14	11	21	.6	23	Trace	.10	.06	.8	Trace
	Italian bread, enriched:																		
331	Loaf, 1 lb——— 1 loaf	454	32	1,250	41	4	.6	.3	1.5	256	77	349	10.0	336	0	1.80	1.10	15.0	0
332	Slice, 4 1/2 by 3 1/4 by 3/4 in.——— 1 slice	30	32	85	3	Trace	Trace	Trace	.1	17	5	23	.7	22	0	.12	.07	1.0	0
	Raisin bread, enriched: [18]																		
333	Loaf, 1 lb——— 1 loaf	454	35	1,190	30	13	3.0	4.7	3.9	243	322	395	10.0	1,057	Trace	1.70	1.07	10.7	Trace
334	Slice (18 per loaf)——— 1 slice	25	35	65	2	1	.2	.3	.2	13	18	22	.6	58	Trace	.09	.06	.6	Trace

Column key (as printed, letters (A)–(S)): (A) Item No. · (B) Food, approximate measure, units, and weight (in grams) · (C) Water (%) · (D) Food energy (cal) · (E) Protein (g) · (F) Fat (g) · (G) Saturated fatty acids (g) · (H) Unsaturated, oleic (g) · (I) Unsaturated, linoleic (g) · (J) Carbohydrate (g) · (K) Calcium (mg) · (L) Phosphorus (mg) · (M) Iron (mg) · (N) Potassium (mg) · (O) Vitamin A (IU) · (P) Thiamin (mg) · (Q) Riboflavin (mg) · (R) Niacin (mg) · (S) Ascorbic acid (mg)

(A)	(B)	(C)	(D)	(E)	(F)	(G)	(H)	(I)	(J)	(K)	(L)	(M)	(N)	(O)	(P)	(Q)	(R)	(S)
	Rye Bread:																	
	American, light (2/3 enriched wheat flour, 1/3 rye flour):																	
335	Loaf, 1 lb — 1 loaf (454 g)	36	1,100	41	5	0.7	0.5	2.2	236	340	667	9.1	658	0	1.35	0.98	12.9	0
336	Slice (4 3/4 by 3 3/4 by 7/16 in) — 1 slice (25 g)	36	60	2	Trace	Trace	Trace	.1	13	19	37	.5	36	0	.07	.05	.7	0
	Pumpernickel (2/3 rye flour, 1/3 enriched wheat flour):																	
337	Loaf, 1 lb — 1 loaf (454 g)	34	1,115	41	5	.7	.5	2.4	241	381	1,039	11.8	2,059	0	1.30	.93	8.5	0
338	Slice (5 by 4 by 3/8 in) — 1 slice (32 g)	34	80	3	Trace	Trace	Trace	.2	17	27	73	.8	145	0	.09	.07	.6	0
	White bread, enriched:[18]																	
	Soft-crumb type:																	
339	Loaf, 1 lb — 1 loaf (454 g)	36	1,225	39	15	3.4	5.3	4.6	229	381	440	11.3	476	Trace	1.80	1.10	15.0	Trace
340	Slice (18 per loaf) — 1 slice (25 g)	36	70	2	1	.2	.3	.3	13	21	24	.6	26	Trace	.10	.06	.8	Trace
341	Slice, toasted — 1 slice (22 g)	25	70	2	1	.2	.3	.3	13	21	24	.6	26	Trace	.08	.06	.8	Trace
342	Slice (22 per loaf) — 1 slice (20 g)	36	55	2	1	.2	.3	.2	10	17	19	.5	21	Trace	.08	.05	.7	Trace
343	Slice, toasted — 1 slice (17 g)	25	55	2	1	.2	.3	.2	10	17	19	.5	21	Trace	.06	.05	.7	Trace
344	Loaf, 1 1/2 lb — 1 loaf (680 g)	36	1,835	59	22	5.2	7.9	6.9	343	571	660	17.0	714	Trace	2.70	1.65	22.5	Trace
345	Slice (24 per loaf) — 1 slice (28 g)	36	75	2	1	.2	.3	.3	14	24	27	.7	29	Trace	.11	.07	.9	Trace
346	Slice, toasted — 1 slice (24 g)	25	75	2	1	.2	.3	.3	14	24	27	.7	29	Trace	.09	.07	.8	Trace
347	Slice (28 per loaf) — 1 slice (24 g)	36	65	2	1	.2	.3	.2	12	20	23	.6	25	Trace	.10	.06	.8	Trace
348	Slice, toasted — 1 slice (21 g)	25	65	2	1	.2	.3	.2	11	20	23	.6	25	Trace	.08	.06	.7	Trace
349	Cubes — 1 cup (30 g)	36	80	3	1	.3	.3	.5	15	25	29	.8	32	Trace	.12	.07	1.0	Trace
350	Crumbs — 1 cup (45 g)	36	120	4	2	.4	.5	.5	23	38	44	1.1	47	Trace	.18	.11	1.5	Trace
	Firm-crumb type:																	
351	Loaf, 1 lb — 1 loaf (454 g)	35	1,245	41	17	3.9	5.9	5.2	228	435	463	11.3	549	Trace	1.80	1.10	15.0	Trace
352	Slice (20 per loaf) — 1 slice (23 g)	35	65	2	1	.2	.3	.3	12	22	23	.6	28	Trace	.09	.06	.8	Trace
353	Slice, toasted — 1 slice (20 g)	24	65	2	1	.2	.3	.3	12	22	23	.6	28	Trace	.07	.06	.8	Trace
354	Loaf, 2 lb — 1 loaf (907 g)	35	2,495	82	34	7.7	11.8	10.4	455	871	925	22.7	1,097	Trace	3.60	2.20	30.0	Trace
355	Slice (34 per loaf) — 1 slice (27 g)	35	75	2	1	.2	.3	.3	14	26	28	.7	33	Trace	.11	.06	.9	Trace
356	Slice, toasted — 1 slice (23 g)	24	75	2	1	.2	.3	.3	14	26	28	.7	33	Trace	.09	.06	.9	Trace
	Whole-wheat bread:																	
	Soft-crumb type:																	
357	Loaf, 1 lb — 1 loaf (454 g)	36	1,095	41	12	2.2	2.9	4.2	224	381	1,152	13.6	1,161	Trace	1.37	.45	12.7	Trace
358	Slice (16 per loaf) — 1 slice (28 g)	36	65	3	1	.1	.2	.2	14	24	71	.8	72	Trace	.09	.03	.8	Trace
359	Slice, toasted — 1 slice (24 g)	24	65	3	1	.1	.2	.2	14	24	71	.8	72	Trace	.07	.03	.8	Trace
	Firm-crumb type:																	
360	Loaf, 1 lb — 1 loaf (454 g)	36	1,100	48	14	2.5	3.3	4.9	216	449	1,034	13.6	1,238	Trace	1.17	.54	12.7	Trace
361	Slice (18 per loaf) — 1 slice (25 g)	36	60	3	1	.1	.2	.2	12	25	57	.8	68	Trace	.06	.03	.7	Trace
362	Slice, toasted — 1 slice (21 g)	24	60	3	1	.1	.2	.3	12	25	57	.8	68	Trace	.05	.03	.7	Trace
	Breakfast cereals:																	
	Hot type, cooked:																	
	Corn (hominy) grits, degermed:																	
363	Enriched — 1 cup (245 g)	87	125	3	Trace	Trace	Trace	—	27	2	25	.7	27	Trace[19]	.10	.07	1.0	0
364	Unenriched — 1 cup (245 g)	87	125	3	Trace	Trace	Trace	—	27	2	25	.2	27	Trace[19]	.05	.02	.5	0
365	Farina, quick-cooking, enriched — 1 cup (245 g)	89	105	3	Trace	Trace	Trace	—	22	147	113[21]	[22]	25	0	.12	.07	1.0	0
366	Oatmeal or rolled oats — 1 cup (240 g)	87	130	5	2	.4	.8	.9	23	22	137	1.4	146	0	.19	.05	.2	0
367	Wheat, rolled — 1 cup (240 g)	80	180	5	1	—	—	—	41	19	182	1.7	202	0	.17	.07	2.2	0
368	Wheat, whole-meal — 1 cup (245 g)	88	110	4	1	—	—	—	23	17	127	1.2	118	0	.15	.05	1.5	0
	Ready-to-eat:																	
369	Bran flakes (40% bran), added sugar, salt, iron, vitamins — 1 cup (35 g)	3	105	4	1	—	—	—	28	19	125	15.6	137	1,650	.41	.49	4.1	12
370	Bran flakes with raisins, added sugar, salt, iron, vitamins — 1 cup (50 g)	7	145	4	1	—	—	—	40	28	146	16.9	154	2,350	.58	.71	5.8	18

[17] Weight includes rind and seeds. Without rind and seeds, weight of the edible portion is 426 g.
[18] Made with vegetable shortening.
[19] Applies to product made with white cornmeal. With yellow cornmeal, value is 30 International Units (I.U.).
[20] Applies to white varieties. For yellow varieties, value is 150 International Units (I.U.).
[21] Applies to products that do not contain di-sodium phosphate. If di-sodium phosphate is an ingredient, value is 162 mg.
[22] Value may range from less than 1 mg to about 8 mg depending on the brand. Consult the label.

GRAIN PRODUCTS—Con.

(A)	(B)		(C)	(D)	(E)	(F)	(G)	(H)	(I)	(J)	(K)	(L)	(M)	(N)	(O)	(P)	(Q)	(R)	(S)
		Grams	Per-cent	Cal-ories	Grams	Grams	Grams	Grams	Grams	Grams	Milli-grams	Milli-grams	Milli-grams	Milli-grams	Inter-national units	Milli-grams	Milli-grams	Milli-grams	Milli-grams
	Breakfast cereals—Continued																		
	Ready-to-eat—Continued																		
	Corn flakes:																		
371	Plain, added sugar, salt, iron, vitamins. 1 cup	25	4	95	2	Trace	—	—	—	21	(**)	9	0.6	30	1,180	0.29	0.35	2.9	9
372	Sugar-coated, added salt, iron, vitamins. 1 cup	40	2	155	2	Trace	—	—	—	37	1	10	1.0	27	1,880	.46	.56	4.6	14
373	Corn, puffed, plain, added sugar, salt, iron, vitamins. 1 cup	20	4	80	2	1	—	—	—	16	4	18	2.3	—	940	.23	.28	2.3	7
374	Corn, shredded, added sugar, salt, iron, thiamin, niacin. 1 cup	25	3	95	2	Trace	—	—	—	22	1	10	.6	—	0	.11	.05	.5	0
375	Oats, puffed, added sugar, salt, minerals, vitamins. 1 cup	25	3	100	3	1	—	—	—	19	44	102	2.9	—	1,180	.29	.35	2.9	9
	Rice, puffed:																		
376	Plain, added iron, thiamin, niacin. 1 cup	15	4	60	1	Trace	—	—	—	13	3	14	.3	15	0	.07	.01	.7	0
377	Presweetened, added salt, iron, vitamins. 1 cup	28	3	115	1	0	—	—	—	26	3	14	**1.1	43	1,250	.38	.43	5.0	*15
378	Wheat flakes, added sugar, salt, iron, vitamins. 1 cup	30	4	105	3	Trace	—	—	—	24	12	83	(**)	81	1,410	.35	.42	3.5	11
	Wheat, puffed:																		
379	Plain, added iron, thiamin, niacin. 1 cup	15	3	55	2	Trace	—	—	—	12	4	48	.6	51	0	.08	.03	1.2	0
380	Presweetened, added salt, iron, vitamins. 1 cup	38	3	140	3	Trace	—	—	—	33	7	52	**1.6	63	1,680	.50	.57	6.7	*20
381	Wheat, shredded, plain. 1 oblong biscuit or 1/2 cup spoon-size biscuits	25	7	90	2	1	—	—	—	20	11	97	.9	87	0	.06	.03	1.1	0
382	Wheat germ, without salt and sugar, toasted. 1 tbsp	6	4	25	2	1	—	—	—	3	3	70	.5	57	10	.11	.05	.3	1
383	Buckwheat flour, light, sifted. 1 cup	98	12	340	6	1	0.2	0.4	0.4	78	11	86	1.0	314	0	.08	.04	.4	0
384	Bulgur, canned, seasoned. 1 cup	135	56	245	8	4	—	—	—	44	27	263	1.9	151	0	.08	.05	4.1	0
	Cake icings. See Sugars and Sweets (items 532-536).																		
	Cakes made from cake mixes with enriched flour:[4]																		
	Angelfood:																		
385	Whole cake (9 3/4-in diam). 1 cake	635	34	1,645	36	1	—	—	—	377	603	756	2.5	381	0	.37	.95	3.6	0
386	Piece, 1/12 of cake (tube cake). 1 piece	53	34	135	3	Trace	—	—	—	32	50	63	.2	32	0	.03	.08	.3	0
	Coffeecake:																		
387	Whole cake (7 3/4 by 5 5/8 by 1 1/4 in). 1 cake	430	30	1,385	27	41	11.7	16.3	8.8	225	262	748	6.9	469	690	.82	.91	7.7	1
388	Piece, 1/6 of cake. 1 piece	72	30	230	5	7	2.0	2.7	1.5	38	44	125	1.2	78	120	.14	.15	1.3	Trace
	Cupcakes, made with egg, milk, 2 1/2-in diam.:																		
389	Without icing. 1 cupcake	25	26	90	1	3	.8	1.2	.7	14	40	59	.3	21	40	.05	.05	.4	Trace
390	With chocolate icing. 1 cupcake	36	22	130	2	5	2.0	1.6	.6	21	47	71	.4	42	60	.05	.06	.4	Trace
	Devil's food with chocolate icing:																		
391	Whole, 2 layer cake (8- or 9-in diam.). 1 cake	1,107	24	3,755	49	136	50.0	44.9	17.0	645	653	1,162	16.6	1,439	1,660	1.06	1.65	10.1	1
392	Piece, 1/16 of cake. 1 piece	69	24	235	3	8	3.1	2.8	1.1	40	41	72	1.0	90	100	.07	.10	.6	Trace
393	Cupcake, 2 1/2-in diam. 1 cupcake	35	24	120	2	4	1.6	1.4	.5	20	21	37	.5	46	50	.03	.05	.3	Trace

		(C)	(D)	(E)	(F)	(G)	(H)	(I)	(J)	(K)	(L)	(M)	(N)	(O)	(P)	(Q)	(R)	(S)
	Gingerbread:																	
394	whole cake (8-in square)——— 1 cake	570	1,575	18	39	9.7	16.6	10.0	291	513	570	8.6	1,562	Trace	0.84	1.00	7.4	Trace
395	Piece, 1/9 of cake——— 1 piece	63	175	2	4	1.1	1.8	1.1	32	57	63	.9	173	Trace	.09	.11	.8	Trace
	White layer cake with chocolate icing:																	
396	Whole cake (8- or 9-in diam.)— 1 cake	1,140	4,000	44	122	48.2	46.4	20.0	716	1,129	2,041	11.4	1,322	680	1.50	1.77	12.5	2
397	Piece, 1/16 of cake——— 1 piece	71	250	3	8	3.0	2.9	1.2	45	70	127	.7	82	40	.09	.11	.8	Trace
	Yellow, 2 layer with chocolate icing:																	
398	whole cake (8- or 9-in diam.)— 1 cake	1,108	3,735	45	125	47.8	47.8	20.3	638	1,008	2,017	12.2	1,208	1,550	1.24	1.67	10.6	2
399	Piece, 1/16 of cake——— 1 piece	69	235	3	8	3.0	3.0	1.3	40	63	126	.8	75	100	.08	.10	.7	Trace
	Cakes made from home recipes using enriched flour:																	
	Boston cream pie with custard filling:																	
400	whole cake (8-in diam.)——— 1 cake	825	2,490	41	78	23.0	30.1	15.2	412	553	833	8.2	*734	1,730	1.04	1.27	9.6	2
401	Piece, 1/12 of cake——— 1 piece	69	210	3	6	1.9	2.5	1.3	34	46	70	.7	*61	140	.09	.11	.8	Trace
	Fruitcake, dark:																	
402	Loaf, 1-lb (7 1/2 by 2 by 1 1/2 in). 1 loaf	454	1,720	22	69	14.4	33.5	14.8	271	327	513	11.8	2,250	540	.72	.73	4.9	2
403	Slice, 1/30 of loaf——— 1 slice	15	55	1	2	.5	1.1	.5	9	11	17	.4	74	20	.02	.02	.2	Trace
	Plain, sheet cake:																	
	Without icing:																	
404	Whole cake (9-in square)——— 1 cake	777	2,830	35	108	29.5	44.4	23.6	434	497	793	8.5	*614	1,320	1.21	1.40	10.2	2
405	Piece, 1/9 of cake——— 1 piece	86	315	4	12	3.3	4.9	2.6	48	55	88	.9	*68	150	.13	.15	1.1	Trace
	With uncooked white icing:																	
406	Whole cake (9-in square)——— 1 cake	1,096	4,020	37	129	42.2	49.5	24.4	694	548	822	8.2	*669	2,190	1.22	1.47	10.2	2
407	Piece, 1/9 of cake——— 1 piece	121	445	4	14	4.7	5.5	2.7	77	61	91	.9	*74	240	.14	.16	1.1	Trace
	Pound:																	
408	Loaf, 8 1/2 by 3 1/2 by 3 1/4 in. 1 loaf	565	2,725	31	170	42.9	73.1	39.6	273	107	418	7.9	345	1,410	.90	.99	7.3	0
409	Slice, 1/17 of loaf——— 1 slice	33	160	2	10	2.5	4.3	2.3	16	6	24	.5	20	80	.05	.06	.4	0
	Spongecake:																	
410	Whole cake (9 3/4-in diam. tube cake). 1 cake	790	2,345	60	45	13.1	15.8	5.7	427	237	885	13.4	687	3,560	1.10	1.64	7.4	Trace
411	Piece, 1/12 of cake——— 1 piece	66	195	5	4	1.1	1.3	.5	36	20	74	1.1	57	300	.09	.14	.6	Trace
	Cookies made with enriched flour:																	
	Brownies with nuts:																	
	Home-prepared, 1 3/4 by 1 3/4 by 7/8 in:																	
412	From home recipe——— 1 brownie	20	95	1	6	1.5	3.0	1.2	10	8	30	.4	38	40	.04	.03	.2	Trace
413	From commercial recipe——— 1 brownie	20	85	1	4	.9	1.4	1.3	13	9	27	.4	34	20	.03	.02	.2	Trace
414	Frozen, with chocolate icing, 1 1/2 by 1 3/4 by 7/8 in. 1 brownie	25	105	1	5	2.0	2.2	.7	15	10	31	.4	44	50	.03	.03	.2	Trace
	Chocolate chip:																	
415	Commercial, 2 1/4-in diam., 3/8 in thick. 4 cookies	42	200	2	9	2.8	2.9	2.2	29	16	48	1.0	56	50	.10	.17	.9	Trace
416	From home recipe, 2 1/3-in diam. 4 cookies	40	205	2	12	3.5	4.5	2.9	24	14	40	.8	47	40	.06	.06	.5	Trace
417	Fig bars, square (1 5/8 by 1 5/8 by 3/8 in) or rectangular 4 cookies	56	200	2	3	.8	1.8	.7	42	44	34	1.0	111	60	.04	.14	.9	Trace
418	Gingersnaps, 2-in diam., 1/4 in thick. 4 cookies	28	90	2	2	.7	1.0	.6	22	20	13	.7	129	20	.08	.06	.7	0
419	Macaroons, 2 3/4-in diam., 1/4 in thick. 2 cookies	38	180	2	9	—	—	—	25	10	32	.3	176	0	.02	.06	.2	0
420	Oatmeal with raisins, 2 5/8-in diam., 1/4 in thick. 4 cookies	52	235	3	8	2.0	3.3	2.0	38	11	53	1.4	192	30	.15	.10	1.0	Trace

Value varies with the brand. Consult the label.
Value varies with the brand. Consult the label.
Applies to product with added ascorbic acid. Without added ascorbic acid, value is trace.
Applies to product with added ascorbic acid.
Excepting angelfood cake, cakes were made from mixes containing vegetable shortening; icings, with butter.
Excepting spongecake, vegetable shortening used for cake portion; butter, for icing. If butter or margarine used for cake portion, vitamin A values would be higher.
Applies to product made with a sodium aluminum-sulfate type baking powder. With a low-sodium type baking powder containing potassium, value would be about twice the amount shown.
Equal weights of flour, sugar, eggs, and vegetable shortening.
Products are commercial unless otherwise specified.
Made with enriched flour and vegetable shortening except for macaroons which do not contain enriched flour or shortening.
Icing made with butter.

(A)	(B) GRAIN PRODUCTS—Con.		(C) Per-cent	(D) Cal-ories	(E) Grams	(F) Grams	(G) Grams	(H) Grams	(I) Grams	(J) Grams	(K) Milli-grams	(L) Milli-grams	(M) Milli-grams	(N) Milli-grams	(O) Inter-national units	(P) Milli-grams	(Q) Milli-grams	(R) Milli-grams	(S) Milli-grams
	Cookies made with enriched flour⁵¹—Continued	Grams																	
421	Plain, prepared from commercial chilled dough, 2 1/2-in diam., 1/4 in. thick.	4 cookies	48	5	240	2	12	3.0	5.2	2.9	31	17	35	0.6	23	30	0.10	0.08	0.9	0
422	Sandwich type (chocolate or vanilla), 1 3/4-in diam., 3/8 in. thick.	4 cookies	40	2	200	2	9	2.2	3.9	2.2	28	10	96	.7	15	0	.06	.10	.7	0
423	Vanilla wafers, 1 3/4-in diam., 1/4 in. thick.	10 cookies	40	3	185	2	6	—	—	—	30	16	25	.6	29	50	.10	.09	.8	0
	Cornmeal:																		
424	Whole-ground, unbolted, dry form.	1 cup	122	12	435	11	5	.5	1.0	2.5	90	24	312	2.9	346	[53]620	.46	.13	2.4	0
425	Bolted (nearly whole-grain), dry form.	1 cup	122	12	440	11	4	.5	.9	2.1	91	21	272	2.2	303	[53]590	.37	.10	2.3	0
	Degermed, enriched:																		
426	Dry form	1 cup	138	12	500	11	2	.2	.4	.9	108	8	137	4.0	166	[53]610	.61	.36	4.8	0
427	Cooked	1 cup	240	88	120	3	Trace	Trace	.1	.2	26	2	34	1.0	38	[53]140	.14	.10	1.2	0
	Degermed, unenriched:																		
428	Dry form	1 cup	138	12	500	11	2	.2	.4	.9	108	8	137	1.5	166	[53]610	.19	.07	1.4	0
429	Cooked	1 cup	240	88	120	3	Trace	Trace	.1	.2	26	2	34	.5	38	[53]140	.05	.02	.2	0
	Crackers:⁵⁰																		
430	Graham, plain, 2 1/2-in square	2 crackers	14	6	55	1	1	.3	.5	.3	10	6	21	.5	55	0	.02	.08	.5	0
431	Rye wafers, whole-grain, 1 7/8 by 3 1/2 in.	2 wafers	13	6	45	2	Trace	—	—	—	10	7	50	.5	78	0	.04	.03	.2	0
432	Saltines, made with enriched flour.	4 crackers or 1 packet	11	4	50	1	1	.3	.5	.4	8	2	10	.5	13	0	.05	.05	.4	0
	Danish pastry (enriched flour), plain without fruit or nuts:⁵⁵																		
433	Packaged ring, 12 oz	1 ring	340	22	1,435	25	80	24.3	31.7	16.5	155	170	371	6.1	381	1,050	.97	1.01	8.6	Trace
434	Round piece, about 4 1/4-in diam. by 1 in.	1 pastry	65	22	275	5	15	4.7	6.1	3.2	30	33	71	1.2	73	200	.18	.19	1.7	Trace
435	Ounce	1 oz	28	22	120	2	7	2.0	2.7	1.4	13	14	31	.5	32	90	.08	.08	.7	Trace
	Doughnuts, made with enriched flour:⁵⁶																		
436	Cake type, plain, 2 1/2-in diam., 1 in. high.	1 doughnut	25	24	100	1	5	1.2	2.0	1.1	13	10	48	.4	23	20	.05	.05	.4	Trace
437	Yeast-leavened, glazed, 3 3/4-in diam., 1 1/4 in. high.	1 doughnut	50	26	205	3	11	3.3	5.8	3.3	22	16	33	.6	34	25	.10	.10	.8	0
	Macaroni, enriched, cooked (cut lengths, elbows, shells):																		
438	Firm stage (hot)	1 cup	130	64	190	7	1	—	—	—	39	14	85	1.4	103	0	.23	.13	1.8	0
	Tender stage:																		
439	Cold macaroni	1 cup	105	73	115	4	Trace	—	—	—	24	8	53	.9	64	0	.15	.08	1.2	0
440	Hot macaroni	1 cup	140	73	155	5	1	—	—	—	32	11	70	1.3	85	0	.20	.11	1.5	0
	Macaroni (enriched) and cheese:																		
441	Canned⁵⁷	1 cup	240	80	230	9	10	4.2	3.1	1.4	26	199	182	1.0	139	260	.12	.24	1.0	Trace
442	From home recipe⁵⁸	1 cup	200	58	430	17	22	8.9	8.8	2.9	40	362	322	1.8	240	860	.20	.40	1.8	Trace
	Muffins made with enriched flour:⁵⁸ From home recipe:																		
443	Blueberry, 2 3/8-in diam., 1 1/2 in. high.	1 muffin	40	39	110	3	4	1.1	1.4	.7	17	34	53	.6	46	90	.09	.10	.7	Trace
444	Bran	1 muffin	40	35	105	3	4	1.2	1.4	.8	17	57	162	1.5	172	90	.07	.10	1.7	Trace
445	Corn (enriched degermed cornmeal and flour), 2 3/8-in diam., 1 1/2 in. high.	1 muffin	40	33	125	3	4	1.2	1.6	.9	19	42	68	.7	54	[57]120	.10	.10	.7	Trace

(A)	(B)		(C)	(D)		(E)	(F)	(G)	(H)	(I)	(J)	(K)	(L)	(M)		(N)	(P)	(O)	(R)	(S)
446	Plain, 3-in diam., 1 1/2 in high	1 muffin	40	38	120	3	4	1.0	1.7	1.0	17	42	60	0.6	50	40	0.09	0.12	0.9	Trace
447	From mix, egg, milk: Corn, 2 3/8-in diam., 1 1/2 in high.[5,8]	1 muffin	40	30	130	3	4	1.2	1.7	.7	20	96	152	.6	44	[5,7]100	.08	.09	.7	Trace
448	Noodles (egg noodles), enriched, cooked.	1 cup	160	71	200	7	2	—	—	—	37	16	94	1.4	70	110	.22	.13	1.9	0
449	Noodles, chow mein, canned.	1 cup	45	1	220	6	11	—	—	—	26	—	—	—	—	—	—	—	—	—
450	Pancakes, (4-in diam.):[14] Buckwheat, made from mix (with buckwheat and enriched flours), egg and milk added.	1 cake	27	58	55	2	2	.8	.9	.4	6	59	91	.4	66	60	.04	.05	.2	Trace
	Plain:																			
.51	Made from home recipe using enriched flour.	1 cake	27	50	60	2	2	.5	.8	.5	9	27	38	.4	33	30	.06	.07	.5	Trace
452	Made from mix with enriched flour, egg and milk added.	1 cake	27	51	60	2	2	.7	.7	.3	9	58	70	.3	42	70	.04	.06	.2	Trace
	Pies, piecrust made with enriched flour, vegetable shortening (9-in diam.):																			
	Apple:																			
453	Whole	1 pie	945	48	2,420	21	105	27.0	44.5	25.2	360	76	208	6.6	756	280	1.06	.79	9.3	9
454	Sector, 1/7 of pie	1 sector	135	48	345	3	15	3.9	6.4	3.6	51	11	30	.9	108	40	.15	.11	1.3	2
	Banana cream:																			
455	Whole	1 pie	910	54	2,010	41	85	26.7	33.2	16.2	279	601	746	7.3	1,847	2,280	.77	1.51	7.0	9
456	Sector, 1/7 of pie	1 sector	130	54	285	6	12	3.8	4.7	2.3	40	86	107	1.0	264	330	.11	.22	1.0	1
	Blueberry:																			
457	Whole	1 pie	945	51	2,285	23	102	24.8	43.7	25.1	330	104	217	9.5	614	280	1.03	.80	10.0	28
458	Sector, 1/7 of pie	1 sector	135	51	325	3	15	3.5	6.2	3.6	47	15	31	1.4	88	40	.15	.11	1.4	4
	Cherry:																			
459	Whole	1 pie	945	47	2,465	25	107	28.2	45.0	25.3	363	132	236	6.6	992	4,160	1.09	.84	9.8	Trace
460	Sector, 1/7 of pie	1 sector	135	47	350	4	15	4.0	6.4	3.6	52	19	34	.9	142	590	.16	.12	1.4	Trace
	Custard:																			
461	Whole	1 pie	910	58	1,985	56	101	33.9	38.5	17.5	213	874	1,028	8.2	1,247	2,090	.79	1.92	5.6	0
462	Sector, 1/7 of pie	1 sector	130	58	285	8	14	4.8	5.5	2.5	30	125	147	1.2	178	300	.11	.27	.8	0
	Lemon meringue:																			
463	Whole	1 pie	840	47	2,140	31	86	26.1	33.8	16.4	317	118	412	6.7	420	1,430	.61	.84	5.2	25
464	Sector, 1/7 of pie	1 sector	120	47	305	4	12	3.7	4.8	2.3	45	17	59	1.0	60	200	.09	.12	.7	4
	Mince:																			
465	Whole	1 pie	945	43	2,560	24	109	28.0	45.9	25.2	389	265	359	13.3	1,682	20	.96	.86	9.8	9
466	Sector, 1/7 of pie	1 sector	135	43	365	3	16	4.0	6.6	3.6	56	38	51	1.9	240	Trace	.14	.12	1.4	1
	Peach:																			
467	Whole	1 pie	945	48	2,410	24	101	24.8	43.7	25.1	361	95	274	8.5	1,408	6,900	1.04	.97	14.0	28
468	Sector, 1/7 of pie	1 sector	135	48	345	3	14	3.5	6.2	3.6	52	14	39	1.2	201	990	.15	.14	2.0	4
	Pecan:																			
469	Whole	1 pie	825	20	3,450	42	189	27.8	101.0	44.2	423	388	850	25.6	1,015	1,320	1.80	.95	6.9	Trace
470	Sector, 1/7 of pie	1 sector	118	20	495	6	27	4.0	14.4	6.3	61	55	122	3.7	145	190	.26	.14	1.0	Trace
	Pumpkin:																			
471	Whole	1 pie	910	59	1,920	36	102	37.4	37.5	16.6	223	464	628	7.3	1,456	22,480	.78	1.27	7.0	Trace
472	Sector, 1/7 of pie	1 sector	130	59	275	5	15	5.4	5.4	2.4	32	66	90	1.0	208	3,210	.11	.18	1.0	Trace
473	Piecrust (home recipe) made with enriched flour and vegetable shortening, baked. Pie shell, 9-in diam.	1 pie shell, 9-in diam.	180	15	900	11	60	14.8	26.1	14.9	79	25	90	3.1	89	0	.47	.40	5.0	0
474	Piecrust mix with enriched flour and vegetable shortening, 10-oz pkg. prepared and baked. Piecrust for 2-crust pie, 9-in diam.	Piecrust for 2-crust pie, 9-in diam.	320	19	1,485	20	93	22.7	39.7	23.4	141	131	272	6.1	179	0	1.07	.79	9.9	0

[15] Made with vegetable shortening.
[2] Products are commercial unless otherwise specified.
[5] Made with enriched flour and vegetable shortening except for macaroons which do not contain flour or shortening.
[3] Applies to yellow varieties; white varieties contain only a trace.
[4] Contains vegetable shortening and butter.
[16] Made with corn oil.
[6] Made with regular margarine.
[7] Applies to product made with yellow cornmeal.
[17] Made with enriched degermed cornmeal and enriched flour.

(A)	(B) GRAIN PRODUCTS—Con.		(C)	(D)	(E)	(F)	(G)	(H)	(I)	(I)	(K)	(L)	(M)	(N)	(O)	(P)	(Q)	(R)	(S)
		Grams	Per cent	Cal ories	Grams	Grams	Grams	Grams	Grams	Grams	Milli grams	Milli grams	Milli grams	Milli grams	Inter national units	Milli grams	Milli grams	Milli grams	Milli grams
475	Pizza (cheese) baked, 4 3/4-in sector; 1/8 of 12-in pie.[15] 1 sector	60	45	145	6	4	1.7	1.5	0.6	22	86	89	1.1	67	230	0.16	0.18	1.6	4
	Popcorn, popped:																		
476	Plain, large kernel 1 cup	6	4	25	1	Trace		.1	.2	5	1	17	.2				.01	.1	0
477	With oil (coconut) and salt added, large kernel 1 cup	9	3	40	1	2	1.5	.2	.2	5	1	19	.2				.01	.2	0
478	Sugar coated 1 cup	35	4	135	2	1	.5	.2	.4	30	2	47	.5				.02	.4	0
	Pretzels, made with enriched flour:																		
479	Dutch, twisted, 2 3/4 by 2 5/8 in. 1 pretzel	16	5	60	2	1				12	4	21	.2	21	0	.05	.04	.7	0
480	Thin, twisted, 3 1/4 by 2 1/4 by 1/4 in. 10 pretzels	60	5	235	6	3				46	13	79	.9	78	0	.20	.15	2.5	0
481	Stick, 2 1/4 in long 10 pretzels	3	5	10	Trace	Trace				2	1	4	Trace	4	0	.01	.01	.1	0
	Rice, white, enriched:																		
	Instant, ready-to-serve, hot:																		
482	1 cup	165	73	180	4	Trace	Trace	Trace	Trace	40	5	31	1.3		0	.21	(**)	1.7	0
	Long grain:																		
483	Raw 1 cup	185	12	670	12	1	.2	.2	.2	149	44	174	5.4	170	0	.81	.06	6.5	0
484	Cooked, served hot 1 cup	205	73	225	4	Trace	.1	.1	.1	50	21	57	1.8	57	0	.23	.02	2.1	0
	Parboiled:																		
485	Raw 1 cup	185	10	685	14	1	.2	.1	.2	150	111	370	5.4	278	0	.81	.07	6.5	0
486	Cooked, served hot 1 cup	175	73	185	4	Trace	.1	.1	.1	41	33	100	1.4	75	0	.19	.02	2.1	0
	Rolls, enriched:[32]																		
	Commercial:																		
487	Brown-and-serve (12 per 12-oz pkg.), browned 1 roll	26	27	85	2	2	.4	.4	.5	14	20	23	.5	25	Trace	.10	.06	.9	Trace
488	Cloverleaf or pan, 2 1/2-in diam., 2 in high. 1 roll	28	31	85	2	2	.4	.4	.4	15	21	24	.5	27	Trace	.11	.07	.9	Trace
489	Frankfurter and hamburger (8 per 11 1/2-oz pkg.), 2 in diam. 1 roll	40	31	120	3	2	.5	.5	.6	21	30	34	.8	38	Trace	.16	.10	1.3	Trace
490	Hard, 3 3/4-in diam., 2 in high. 1 roll	50	25	155	5	2	.4	.4	.5	30	24	46	1.2	49	Trace	.20	.12	1.7	Trace
491	Hoagie or submarine, 11 1/2 by 3 by 2 1/2 in. 1 roll	135	31	390	12	4	.9	1.4	1.4	75	58	115	3.0	122	Trace	.54	.32	4.5	Trace
	From home recipe:																		
492	Cloverleaf, 2 1/2-in diam., 2 in high. 1 roll	35	26	120	3	3	.8	1.1	.7	20	16	36	.7	41	30	.12	.12	1.2	Trace
	Spaghetti, enriched, cooked:																		
493	Firm stage, "al dente," served hot 1 cup	130	64	190	7	1				39	14	85	1.4	103	0	.23	.13	1.8	0
494	Tender stage, served hot 1 cup	140	73	155	5	1				32	11	70	1.3	85	0	.20	.11	1.5	0
	Spaghetti (enriched) in tomato sauce with cheese:																		
495	From home recipe 1 cup	250	77	260	9	9	2.0	5.4	.7	37	80	135	2.3	408	1,080	.25	.18	2.3	13
496	Canned 1 cup	250	80	190	6	2	.5	.3	.4	39	40	88	2.8	303	930	.35	.28	4.5	10
	Spaghetti (enriched) with meat balls and tomato sauce:																		
497	From home recipe 1 cup	248	70	330	19	12	3.3	6.3	.9	39	124	236	3.7	665	1,590	.25	.30	4.0	22
498	Canned 1 cup	250	78	260	12	10	2.2	3.3	3.9	29	53	113	3.3	245	1,000	.15	.18	2.3	5
499	Toaster pastries 1 pastry	50	12	200	3	6				36	54	[67]	1.9	[474]	500	.16	.17	2.1	(16)
	Waffles, made with enriched flour, 7-in diam.:[33]																		
500	From home recipe 1 waffle	75	41	210	7	7	2.3	2.8	1.4	28	85	130	1.3	109	250	.17	.23	1.4	Trace
501	From mix, egg and milk added 1 waffle	75	42	205	7	8	2.8	2.9	1.2	27	179	257	1.0	146	170	.14	.22	.9	Trace

(A)	(B)	(C)	(D)	(E)	(F)	(G)	(H)	(I)	(J)	(K)	(L)	(M)	(N)	(O)	(P)	(Q)	(R)	(S)
	Wheat flours:																	
	All-purpose or family flour, enriched:																	
502	Sifted, spooned — 1 cup (115)	12	420	12	1	0.2	0.1	0.5	88	18	100	3.3	109	0	0.74	0.46	6.1	0
503	Unsifted, spooned — 1 cup (125)	12	455	13	1	.2	.1	.5	95	20	109	3.6	119	0	.80	.50	6.6	0
504	Cake or pastry flour, enriched, sifted, spooned — 1 cup (96)	12	350	7	1	.1	.1	.3	76	16	70	2.8	91	0	.61	.38	5.1	0
505	Self-rising, enriched, unsifted, spooned — 1 cup (125)	12	440	12	1	.2	.1	.5	93	331	583	3.6	—	0	.80	.50	6.6	0
506	Whole-wheat, from hard wheats, stirred — 1 cup (120)	12	400	16	2	.4	.2	1.0	85	49	446	4.0	444	0	.66	.14	5.2	0
	LEGUMES (DRY), NUTS, SEEDS; RELATED PRODUCTS																	
	Almonds, shelled:																	
507	Chopped (about 130 almonds) — 1 cup (130)	5	775	24	70	5.6	47.7	12.8	25	304	655	6.1	1,005	0	.31	1.20	4.6	Trace
508	Slivered, not pressed down (about 115 almonds) — 1 cup (115)	5	690	21	62	5.0	42.2	11.3	22	269	580	5.4	889	0	.28	1.06	4.0	Trace
	Beans, dry:																	
	Common varieties as Great Northern, navy, and others:																	
	Cooked, drained:																	
509	Great Northern — 1 cup (180)	69	210	14	1	—	—	—	38	90	266	4.9	749	0	.25	.13	1.3	0
510	Pea (navy) — 1 cup (190)	69	225	15	1	—	—	—	40	95	281	5.1	790	0	.27	.13	1.3	0
	Canned, solids and liquid:																	
	White with—																	
511	Frankfurters (sliced) — 1 cup (255)	71	365	19	18	2.4	2.8	.6	32	94	303	4.8	668	330	.18	.15	3.3	Trace
512	Pork and tomato sauce — 1 cup (255)	71	310	16	7	4.3	5.0	1.1	48	138	235	4.6	536	330	.20	.08	1.5	5
513	Pork and sweet sauce — 1 cup (255)	66	385	16	12	—	—	—	54	161	291	5.9	—	—	.15	.10	1.5	—
514	Red kidney — 1 cup (255)	76	230	15	1	—	—	—	42	74	278	4.6	673	10	.13	.10	1.5	—
515	Lima, cooked, drained — 1 cup (190)	64	260	16	1	—	—	—	49	55	293	5.9	1,163	10	.25	.11	1.3	—
516	Blackeye peas, dry, cooked (with residual cooking liquid) — 1 cup (250)	80	190	13	1	—	—	—	35	43	238	3.3	573	30	.40	.10	1.0	—
517	Brazil nuts, shelled (6-8 large kernels) — 1 oz (28)	5	185	4	19	4.8	6.2	7.1	3	53	196	1.0	203	Trace	.27	.03	.5	—
518	Cashew nuts, roasted in oil — 1 cup (140)	5	785	24	64	12.9	36.8	10.2	41	53	522	5.3	650	140	.60	.35	2.5	—
	Coconut meat, fresh:																	
519	Piece about 2 by 2 by 1/2 in — 1 piece (45)	51	155	2	16	14.0	.9	.9	4	6	43	.8	115	0	.02	.01	.2	1
520	Shredded or grated, not pressed down — 1 cup (80)	51	275	3	28	24.8	1.6	.5	8	10	76	1.4	205	0	.04	.02	.4	2
521	Filberts (hazelnuts), chopped (about 80 kernels) — 1 cup (115)	6	730	14	72	5.1	55.2	7.3	19	240	388	3.9	810	0	.53	—	1.0	Trace
522	Lentils, whole, cooked — 1 cup (200)	72	210	16	Trace	—	—	—	39	50	238	4.2	498	40	.14	.12	1.2	0
523	Peanuts, roasted in oil, salted (whole, halves, chopped) — 1 cup (144)	2	840	37	72	13.7	33.0	20.7	27	107	577	3.0	971	—	.46	.19	24.8	0
524	Peanut butter — 1 tbsp (16)	2	95	4	8	1.5	3.7	2.3	3	9	61	.3	100	—	.02	.02	2.4	0
525	Peas, split, dry, cooked — 1 cup (200)	70	230	16	1	—	—	—	42	22	178	3.4	592	80	.30	.18	1.8	—
526	Pecans, chopped or pieces (about 120 large halves) — 1 cup (118)	3	810	11	84	7.2	50.5	20.0	17	86	341	2.8	712	150	1.01	.15	1.1	2
527	Pumpkin and squash kernels, dry, hulled — 1 cup (140)	4	775	41	65	11.8	23.5	27.5	21	71	1,602	15.7	1,386	100	.34	.27	3.4	—
528	Sunflower seeds, dry, hulled — 1 cup (145)	5	810	35	69	8.2	13.7	43.2	29	174	1,214	10.3	1,334	70	2.84	.33	7.8	—
	Walnuts:																	
	Black:																	
529	Chopped or broken kernels — 1 cup (125)	3	785	26	74	6.3	13.3	45.7	19	Trace	713	7.5	575	380	.28	.14	.9	—
530	Ground (finely) — 1 cup (80)	3	500	16	47	4.0	8.5	29.2	12	Trace	456	4.8	368	240	.18	.09	.6	—
531	Persian or English, chopped (about 60 halves) — 1 cup (120)	4	780	18	77	8.4	11.8	42.2	19	119	456	3.7	540	40	.40	.16	1.1	2

[1] Crust made with vegetable shortening and enriched flour.
[2] Made with vegetable shortening.
[3] Product may or may not be enriched with riboflavin. Consult the label.
[4] Value varies with the brand. Consult the label.

	(B) SUGARS AND SWEETS	Grams	(C) Per-cent	(D) Cal-ories	(E) Grams	(F) Grams	(G) Grams	(H) Grams	(I) Grams	(J) Grams	(K) Milli-grams	(L) Milli-grams	(M) Milli-grams	(N) Milli-grams	(O) Inter-national units	(P) Milli-grams	(Q) Milli-grams	(R) Milli-grams	(S) Milli-grams
	Cake icings: Boiled, white:																		
532	Plain	94	18	295	1	0	0	0	0	75	2	2	Trace	17	0	Trace	0.03	Trace	0
533	With coconut	166	15	605	3	13	11.0	.9	Trace	124	10	50	0.8	277	0	0.02	.07	0.3	0
534	Uncooked: Chocolate made with milk and butter	275	14	1,035	9	38	23.4	11.7	1.0	185	165	305	3.3	536	580	.06	.28	.6	1
535	Creamy fudge from mix and water	245	15	830	7	16	5.1	6.7	3.1	183	96	218	2.7	238	Trace	.05	.20	.7	Trace
536	White	319	11	1,200	2	21	12.7	5.1	.5	260	48	38	Trace	57	860	Trace	.06	.1	Trace
537	Candy: Caramels, plain or chocolate	28	8	115	1	3	1.6	1.1	.1	22	42	35	.4	54	Trace	.01	.05	.1	Trace
	Chocolate:																		
538	Milk, plain	28	1	145	2	9	5.5	3.0	.3	16	65	65	.3	109	80	.02	.10	.1	Trace
539	Semisweet, small pieces (60 per oz)	170	1	860	7	61	36.2	19.8	1.7	97	51	255	4.4	553	30	.02	.14	.9	0
540	Chocolate-coated peanuts	28	1	160	5	12	4.0	4.7	2.1	11	33	84	.4	143	Trace	.10	.05	2.1	Trace
541	Fondant, uncoated (mints, candy corn, other)	28	8	105	Trace	1	.3	.1	.1	25	4	2	.3	1	0	Trace	Trace	Trace	0
542	Fudge, chocolate, plain	28	8	115	1	3	1.3	1.4	.6	21	22	24	.3	42	Trace	.01	.03	.1	Trace
543	Gum drops	28	12	100	Trace	Trace				25	2	Trace	.1	1	0	0	0	Trace	0
544	Hard	28	1	110	0	Trace				28	6	2	.5	1	0	0	0	0	0
545	Marshmallows	28	17	90	1	Trace				23	5	2	.5	2	0	0	Trace	Trace	0
	Chocolate-flavored beverage powders (about 4 heaping tsp per oz):																		
546	With nonfat dry milk	28	2	100	5	1	.5	.3	Trace	20	167	155	.5	227	10	.04	.21	.2	1
547	Without milk	28	1	100	1	1	.4	.2	Trace	25	9	48	.6	142	0	.01	.03	.1	0
548	Honey, strained or extracted	21	17	65	Trace	0				17	1	2	.1	11	Trace	Trace	.01	.1	Trace
549	Jams and preserves	20	29	55	Trace	Trace				14	4	2	.2	18	Trace	Trace	.01	Trace	Trace
550	packet	14	29	40	Trace	Trace				10	3	1	.1	12	Trace	Trace	.01	Trace	Trace
551	Jellies	18	29	50	Trace	Trace				13	4	1	.3	14	Trace	Trace	.01	Trace	Trace
552	packet	14	29	40	Trace	Trace				10	3	1	.2	11	Trace	Trace	Trace	Trace	Trace
	Syrups: Chocolate-flavored sirup or topping:																		
553	Thin type	38	32	90	1	1	.5	.3	Trace	24	6	35	.6	106	Trace	.01	.03	.2	0
554	Fudge type	38	25	125	2	5	3.1	1.6	.1	20	48	60	.5	107	60	.02	.08	.2	Trace
	Molasses, cane:																		
555	Light (first extraction)	20	24	50						13	33	9	.9	183		.01	.01	Trace	
556	Blackstrap (third extraction)	20	24	45						11	137	17	3.2	585		.02	.04	.4	
557	Sorghum	21	23	55						14	35	5	2.6			.02	.02	Trace	
558	Table blends, chiefly corn, light and dark	21	24	60	0	0				15	9	3	.8	1	0	0	0	0	0
	Sugars:																		
559	Brown, pressed down	220	2	820	0	0				212	187	42	7.5	757	0	.02	.07	.4	0
	White:																		
560	Granulated	200	1	770	0	0				199	0	0	.2	6	0	0	0	0	0
561	tbsp	12	1	45	0	0				12	0	0	Trace	Trace	0	0	0	0	0
562	packet	6	1	23	0	0				6	0	0	Trace	Trace	0	0	0	0	0
563	Powdered, sifted, spooned into cup.	100	1	385	0	0				100	0	0	.1	3	0	0	0	0	0

VEGETABLE AND VEGETABLE PRODUCTS

(A)	(B)	(C)	(D)	(E)	(F)	(G)	(H)	(I)	(J)	(K)	(L)	(M)	(N)	(O)	(P)	(Q)	(R)	(S)
	Asparagus, green: Cooked, drained: Cuts and tips, 1 1/2- to 2-in lengths:																	
564	From raw------ 1 cup	145	94	30	3	Trace	—	—	—	2	5	30	73	0.9	265	1,310	0.23	0.26	2.0	38
565	From frozen------ 1 cup	180	93	40	6	Trace	—	—	—	2	6	40	115	2.2	396	1,530	.25	.23	1.8	41
	Spears, 1/2-in diam. at base:																	
566	From raw------ 4 spears	60	94	10	1	Trace	—	—	—	2	13	13	30	.4	110	540	.10	.11	.8	16
567	From frozen------ 4 spears	60	92	15	2	Trace	—	—	—	2	13	13	40	.7	143	470	.10	.08	.7	16
568	Canned, spears, 1/2-in diam. at base.------ 4 spears	80	93	15	2	Trace	—	—	—	3	15	15	42	1.5	133	640	.05	.08	.6	12
	Beans: Lima, immature seeds, frozen, cooked, drained:																	
569	Thick-seeded types (Fordhooks)-- 1 cup	170	74	170	10	Trace	—	—	—	32	32	34	153	2.9	724	390	.12	.09	1.7	29
570	Thin-seeded types (baby limas)-- 1 cup	180	69	210	13	Trace	—	—	—	40	40	63	227	4.7	709	400	.16	.09	2.2	22
	Snap: Green: Cooked, drained:																	
571	From raw (cuts and French style)-- 1 cup	125	92	30	2	Trace	—	—	—	7	7	63	46	.8	189	680	.09	.11	.6	15
	From frozen:																	
572	Cuts------ 1 cup	135	92	35	2	Trace	—	—	—	8	8	54	43	.9	205	780	.09	.12	.5	7
573	French style------ 1 cup	130	92	35	2	Trace	—	—	—	8	8	49	39	1.2	177	690	.08	.10	.4	9
574	Canned, drained solids (cuts)-- 1 cup	135	92	30	2	Trace	—	—	—	7	7	61	34	2.0	128	630	.04	.07	.4	5
	Yellow or wax: Cooked, drained:																	
575	From raw (cuts and French style)-- 1 cup	125	93	30	2	Trace	—	—	—	6	6	63	46	.8	189	290	.09	.11	.6	16
576	From frozen (cuts)-- 1 cup	135	92	35	2	Trace	—	—	—	8	8	47	42	.9	221	140	.09	.11	.5	8
577	Canned, drained solids (cuts)-- 1 cup	135	92	30	2	Trace	—	—	—	7	7	61	34	2.0	128	140	.04	.07	.4	7
	Beans, mature. See Beans, dry (items 509-515) and Blackeye peas, dry (item 516). Bean sprouts (mung):																	
578	Raw------ 1 cup	105	89	35	4	Trace	—	—	—	7	7	20	67	1.4	234	20	.14	.14	.8	20
579	Cooked, drained------ 1 cup	125	91	35	4	Trace	—	—	—	7	7	21	60	1.1	195	30	.11	.13	.9	8
	Beets: Cooked, drained, peeled:																	
580	Whole beets, 2-in diam.-- 2 beets	100	91	30	1	Trace	—	—	—	7	7	14	23	.5	208	20	.03	.04	.3	6
581	Diced or sliced------ 1 cup	170	91	55	2	Trace	—	—	—	12	12	24	39	.9	354	30	.05	.07	.5	10
	Canned, drained solids:																	
582	Whole beets, small------ 1 cup	160	89	60	1	Trace	—	—	—	14	14	30	29	1.1	267	20	.02	.05	.2	5
583	Diced or sliced------ 1 cup	170	89	65	2	Trace	—	—	—	15	15	32	31	1.2	284	30	.02	.05	.2	5
584	Beet greens, leaves and stems, cooked, drained.-- 1 cup	145	94	25	2	Trace	—	—	—	5	5	144	36	2.8	481	7,400	.10	.22	.4	22
	Blackeye peas, immature seeds, cooked and drained:																	
585	From raw------ 1 cup	165	72	180	13	1	—	—	—	30	30	40	241	3.5	625	580	.50	.18	2.3	28
586	From frozen------ 1 cup	170	66	220	15	1	—	—	—	40	40	43	286	4.8	573	290	.68	.19	2.4	15
	Broccoli, cooked, drained: From raw:																	
587	Stalk, medium size------ 1 stalk	180	91	45	6	1	—	—	—	8	8	158	112	1.4	481	4,500	.16	.36	1.4	162
588	Stalks cut into 1/2-in pieces-- 1 cup	155	91	40	5	Trace	—	—	—	7	7	136	96	1.2	414	3,880	.14	.31	1.2	140
	From frozen:																	
589	Stalk, 4 1/2 to 5 in long-- 1 stalk	30	91	10	1	Trace	—	—	—	1	1	12	17	.2	66	570	.02	.03	.2	22
590	Chopped------ 1 cup	185	92	50	5	1	—	—	—	9	9	100	104	1.3	392	4,810	.11	.22	.9	105
591	Brussels sprouts, cooked, drained: From raw, 7-8 sprouts (1 1/4- to 1 1/2-in diam.).-- 1 cup	155	88	55	7	1	—	—	—	10	10	50	112	1.7	423	810	.12	.22	1.2	135
592	From frozen------ 1 cup	155	89	50	5	Trace	—	—	—	10	10	33	95	1.2	457	880	.12	.16	.9	126

VEGETABLE AND VEGETABLE PRODUCTS—Con.

No. (A)	Food (B)	Grams	(C) Per cent	(D) Calories	(E) Grams	(F) Grams	(G) Grams	(H) Grams	(I) Grams	(I) Grams	(K) Milligrams	(L) Milligrams	(M) Milligrams	(N) Milligrams	(O) International units	(P) Milligrams	(Q) Milligrams	(R) Milligrams	(S) Milligrams
	Cabbage:																		
	Common varieties:																		
	Raw:																		
593	Coarsely shredded or sliced—— 1 cup	70	92	15	1	Trace	—	—	—	4	34	20	0.3	163	90	0.04	0.04	.2	33
594	Finely shredded or chopped—— 1 cup	90	92	20	1	Trace	—	—	—	5	44	26	.4	210	120	.05	.05	.3	42
595	Cooked, drained—— 1 cup	145	94	30	2	Trace	—	—	—	6	64	29	.4	236	190	.06	.06	.4	48
596	Red, raw, coarsely shredded or sliced. 1 cup	70	90	20	1	Trace	—	—	—	5	29	25	.6	188	30	.06	.04	.3	43
597	Savoy, raw, coarsely shredded or sliced. 1 cup	70	92	15	2	Trace	—	—	—	3	47	38	.6	188	140	.04	.06	.2	39
598	Cabbage, celery (also called pe-tsai or wongbok), raw, 1-in pieces—— 1 cup	75	95	10	1	Trace	—	—	—	2	32	30	.5	190	110	.04	.03	.5	19
599	Cabbage, white mustard (also called bokchoy or pakchoy), cooked, drained—— 1 cup	170	95	25	2	Trace	—	—	—	4	252	56	1.0	364	5,270	.07	.14	1.2	26
	Carrots:																		
	Raw, without crowns and tips, scraped:																		
600	Whole, 7 1/2 by 1 1/8 in, or strips, 2 1/2 to 3 in long—— 1 carrot or 18 strips	72	88	30	1	Trace	—	—	—	7	27	26	.5	246	7,930	.04	.04	.4	6
601	Grated—— 1 cup	110	88	45	1	Trace	—	—	—	11	41	40	.8	375	12,100	.07	.06	.7	9
602	Cooked (crosswise cuts), drained—— 1 cup	155	91	50	1	Trace	—	—	—	11	51	48	.9	344	16,280	.08	.08	.8	9
	Canned:																		
603	Sliced, drained solids—— 1 cup	155	91	45	1	Trace	—	—	—	10	47	34	1.1	186	23,250	.03	.05	.6	3
604	Strained or Junior (baby food)—— 1 oz (1 3/4 to 2 tbsp)	28	92	10	Trace	Trace	—	—	—	2	7	6	.1	51	3,690	.01	.01	.1	1
	Cauliflower:																		
605	Raw, chopped—— 1 cup	115	91	31	3	Trace	—	—	—	6	29	64	1.3	339	70	.13	.12	.8	90
	Cooked, drained:																		
606	From raw (flower buds)—— 1 cup	125	93	30	3	Trace	—	—	—	5	26	53	.9	258	80	.11	.10	.8	69
607	From frozen (flowerets)—— 1 cup	180	94	30	3	Trace	—	—	—	6	31	68	.9	373	50	.07	.09	.7	74
	Celery, Pascal type, raw:																		
608	Stalk, large outer, 8 by 1 1/2 in, at root end.—— 1 stalk	40	94	5	Trace	Trace	—	—	—	2	16	11	.1	136	110	.01	.01	.1	4
609	Pieces, diced—— 1 cup	120	94	20	1	Trace	—	—	—	5	47	34	.4	409	320	.04	.04	.4	11
	Collards, cooked, drained:																		
610	From raw (leaves without stems)—— 1 cup	190	90	65	7	1	—	—	—	10	357	99	1.5	498	14,820	.21	.38	2.3	144
611	From frozen (chopped)—— 1 cup	170	90	50	5	1	—	—	—	10	299	87	1.7	401	11,560	.10	.24	1.0	56
	Corn, sweet:																		
	Cooked, drained:																		
612	From raw, ear 5 by 1 3/4 in—— 1 ear	140	74	70	2	1	—	—	—	16	2	69	.5	151	[4]310	.09	.08	1.1	7
	From frozen:																		
613	Ear, 5 in long—— 1 ear	229	73	120	4	1	—	—	—	27	4	121	1.0	291	[4]440	.18	.10	2.1	9
614	Kernels—— 1 cup	165	77	130	5	1	—	—	—	31	5	120	1.3	304	[4]580	.15	.10	2.5	8
	Canned:																		
615	Cream style—— 1 cup	256	76	210	5	2	—	—	—	51	8	143	1.5	248	[4]840	.08	.13	2.6	13
	Whole kernel:																		
616	Wet pack, drained solids—— 1 cup	210	76	175	5	1	—	—	—	43	6	153	1.1	204	[6]740	.06	.13	2.3	11
617	Vacuum pack—— 1 cup	165	76	140	4	1	—	—	—	33	8	81	.8	160	[6]580	.05	.08	1.5	7
	Cowpeas. See Blackeye peas. (Items 585-586).																		
	Cucumber slices, 1/8 in thick (large, 2 1/8-in diam.; small, 1 3/4-in diam.):																		
618	With peel—— 6 large or 8 small slices	28	95	5	Trace	Trace	—	—	—	1	7	8	.3	45	70	.01	.01	.1	3

Table of nutritive values of foods (items 619–651). Columns are lettered (B)–(S): (B) food and approximate measure; grams; (C) water %; (D) food energy; (E) protein; (F) fat; (G) saturated, (H) oleic, (I) linoleic fatty acids; (J) carbohydrate; (K) calcium; (L) phosphorus; (M) iron; (N) potassium; (O) vitamin A; (P) thiamin; (Q) riboflavin; (R) niacin; (S) ascorbic acid.

No.	(B) Food, approximate measure	g	(C)	(D)	(E)	(F)	(G)	(H)	(I)	(J)	(K)	(L)	(M)	(N)	(O)	(P)	(Q)	(R)	(S)
619	Without peel — 6 1/2 large or 9 small pieces	28	96	5	Trace	Trace	—	—	—	1	7	7	.1	45	Trace	.01	.01	.1	3
620	Dandelion greens, cooked, drained — 1 cup	105	90	35	2	Trace	—	—	—	7	147	44	1.9	244	12,290	.14	.17	—	19
621	Endive, curly (including escarole), raw, small pieces — 1 cup	50	93	10	1	Trace	—	—	—	2	41	27	.9	147	1,650	.04	.07	.3	5
622	Kale, cooked, drained: From raw (leaves without stems and midribs) — 1 cup	110	88	45	5	1	—	—	—	7	206	64	1.8	243	9,130	.11	.20	1.8	102
623	From frozen (leaf style) — 1 cup	130	91	40	4	1	—	—	—	7	157	62	1.3	251	10,660	.08	.20	.9	49
	Lettuce, raw:																		
624	Butterhead, as Boston types: Head, 5-in diam — 1 head	220	95	25	2	Trace	—	—	—	4	57	42	3.3	430	1,580	.10	.10	.3	13
625	Leaves — 1 outer or 2 inner or 3 heart leaves	15	95	Trace	Trace	Trace	—	—	—	Trace	5	4	.3	40	150	.01	.01	Trace	1
626	Crisphead, as Iceberg: Head, 6-in diam — 1 head	567	96	70	5	1	—	—	—	16	108	118	2.7	943	1,780	.32	.32	1.6	32
627	Wedge, 1/4 of head — 1 wedge	135	96	20	1	Trace	—	—	—	4	27	30	.7	236	450	.08	.08	.4	8
628	Pieces, chopped or shredded — 1 cup	55	96	5	Trace	Trace	—	—	—	2	11	12	.3	96	180	.03	.03	.2	3
629	Looseleaf (bunching varieties including romaine or cos), chopped or shredded pieces — 1 cup	55	94	10	1	Trace	—	—	—	2	37	14	.8	145	1,050	.03	.04	.2	10
630	Mushrooms, raw, sliced or chopped pieces — 1 cup	70	90	20	2	Trace	—	—	—	3	4	81	.6	290	Trace	.07	.32	2.9	2
631	Mustard greens, without stems and midribs; cooked, drained — 1 cup	140	93	30	3	1	—	—	—	6	193	45	2.5	308	8,120	.11	.20	.8	67
632	Okra pods, 3 by 5/8 in, cooked — 10 pods	106	91	30	2	Trace	—	—	—	6	98	43	.5	184	520	.14	.19	1.0	21
	Onions: Mature: Raw:																		
633	Chopped — 1 cup	170	89	65	3	Trace	—	—	—	15	46	61	.9	267	Trace	.05	.07	.2	17
634	Sliced — 1 cup	115	89	45	2	Trace	—	—	—	10	31	41	.6	181	Trace	.03	.05	.1	12
635	Cooked (whole or sliced), drained — 1 cup	210	92	60	3	Trace	—	—	—	14	50	61	.8	231	Trace	.06	.06	.2	15
636	Young green, bulb (3/8 in diam.) and white portion of top — 6 onions	30	88	15	Trace	Trace	—	—	—	3	12	12	.2	69	Trace	.02	.01	.1	8
637	Parsley, raw, chopped — 1 tbsp	4	85	Trace	Trace	Trace	—	—	—	Trace	7	2	.2	25	300	Trace	.01	.1	6
638	Parsnips, cooked (diced or 2-in lengths) — 1 cup	155	82	100	2	1	—	—	—	23	70	96	.9	587	50	.11	.12	.2	16
	Peas, green:																		
639	Canned: drained solids — 1 cup	170	77	150	8	1	—	—	—	29	44	129	3.2	163	1,170	.15	.10	1.4	14
640	Strained (baby food) — 1 oz (1 3/4 to 2 tbsp)	28	86	15	1	Trace	—	—	—	3	3	18	.3	28	140	.02	.03	.3	3
641	Frozen, cooked, drained — 1 cup	160	85	110	8	1	—	—	—	19	30	138	3.0	216	960	.43	.14	2.7	21
642	Peppers, hot, red, without seeds, dried (ground chili powder, added seasonings) — 1 tsp	2	9	5	Trace	Trace	—	—	—	1	5	4	.4	20	1,300	Trace	.02	.2	Trace
	Peppers, sweet (about 5 per lb, stems and seeds removed):																		
643	Raw — 1 pod	74	93	15	1	Trace	—	—	—	4	7	16	.5	157	310	.06	.06	.4	94
644	Cooked, boiled, drained — 1 pod	73	95	15	1	Trace	—	—	—	3	7	12	.4	109	310	.05	.05	.4	70
645	Potatoes, cooked: Baked, peeled after baking (about 2 per lb, raw) — 1 potato	156	75	145	4	Trace	—	—	—	33	14	101	1.1	782	Trace	.15	.07	2.7	31
	Boiled (about 3 per lb, raw):																		
646	Peeled after boiling — 1 potato	137	80	105	3	Trace	—	—	—	23	10	72	.8	556	Trace	.12	.05	2.0	22
647	Peeled before boiling — 1 potato	135	83	90	3	Trace	—	—	—	20	8	57	.7	385	Trace	.12	.05	1.6	22
	French-fried, strip, 2 to 3 1/2 in long:																		
648	Prepared from raw — 10 strips	50	45	135	2	7	1.7	1.2	3.3	18	8	56	.7	427	Trace	.07	.04	1.6	11
649	Frozen, oven heated — 10 strips	50	53	110	2	4	1.1	.8	2.1	17	5	43	.9	326	Trace	.07	.01	1.3	11
650	Hashed brown, prepared from frozen — 1 cup	155	56	345	3	18	4.6	3.2	9.0	45	28	78	1.9	439	Trace	.11	.03	1.6	12
	Mashed, prepared from: Raw:																		
651	Milk added — 1 cup	210	83	135	4	2	.7	.4	Trace	27	50	103	.8	548	40	.17	.11	2.1	21

¹Weight includes cob. Without cob, weight is 77 g for item 612, 126 g for item 613.
²Based on yellow varieties. For white varieties, value is trace.
³Weight includes refuse of outer leaves and core. Without these parts, weight is 163 g.
⁴Weight includes core. Without core, weight is 539 g.
⁵Value based on white-fleshed varieties. For yellow-fleshed varieties, value in International Units (I.U.) is 70 for item 633, 50 for item 634, and 80 for item 635.

VEGETABLE AND VEGETABLE PRODUCTS—Con.

(A) No.	(B) Food, approximate measure	(C) Grams	(D) Water %	(E) Calories	(F) Protein (g)	(G) Fat (g)	(H) Saturated (g)	(I) Oleic (g)	(J) Linoleic (g)	(K) Carbohydrate (g)	(L) Calcium (mg)	(M) Phosphorus (mg)	(N) Iron (mg)	(O) Potassium (mg)	(P) Vitamin A (IU)	(Q) Thiamin (mg)	(R) Riboflavin (mg)	(S) Niacin (mg)	(T) Ascorbic acid (mg)
	Potatoes, cooked—Continued																		
	Mashed, prepared from—Continued																		
	Raw—Continued																		
652	Milk and butter added — 1 cup	210	80	195	4	9	5.6	2.3	0.2	26	50	101	0.8	525	360	0.17	0.11	2.1	19
653	Dehydrated flakes (without milk), water, milk, butter, and salt added — 1 cup	210	79	195	4	7	3.6	2.1	.2	30	65	99	.6	601	270	.08	.08	1.9	11
654	Potato chips, 1 3/4 by 2 1/2 in oval cross section — 10 chips	20	2	115	1	8	2.1	1.4	4.0	10	8	28	.4	226	Trace	.04	.01	1.0	3
655	Potato salad, made with cooked salad dressing — 1 cup	250	76	250	7	7	2.0	2.7	1.3	41	80	160	1.5	798	350	.20	.18	2.8	28
656	Pumpkin, canned — 1 cup	245	90	80	2	1	—	—	—	19	61	64	1.0	588	15,680	.07	.12	1.5	12
657	Radishes, raw (prepackaged) stem ends, rootlets cut off — 4 radishes	18	95	5	Trace	Trace	—	—	—	1	5	6	.2	58	Trace	.01	.01	.1	5
658	Sauerkraut, canned, solids and liquid — 1 cup	235	93	40	2	Trace	—	—	—	9	85	42	1.2	329	120	.07	.09	.5	33
	Southern peas. See Blackeye peas (items 585-586).																		
	Spinach:																		
659	Raw, chopped — 1 cup	55	91	15	2	Trace	—	—	—	2	51	28	1.7	259	4,460	.06	.11	.3	28
660	Cooked, drained: From raw — 1 cup	180	92	40	5	1	—	—	—	6	167	68	4.0	583	14,580	.13	.25	.9	50
	From frozen:																		
661	Chopped — 1 cup	205	92	45	6	1	—	—	—	8	232	90	4.3	683	16,200	.14	.31	.8	39
662	Leaf — 1 cup	190	92	45	6	1	—	—	—	7	200	84	4.8	688	15,390	.15	.27	1.0	53
663	Canned, drained solids — 1 cup	205	91	50	6	1	—	—	—	7	242	53	5.3	513	16,400	.04	.25	.6	29
	Squash, cooked:																		
664	Summer (all varieties), diced, drained — 1 cup	210	96	30	2	Trace	—	—	—	7	53	53	.8	296	820	.11	.17	1.7	21
665	Winter (all varieties), baked, mashed — 1 cup	205	81	130	4	1	—	—	—	32	57	98	1.6	945	8,610	.10	.27	1.4	27
	Sweetpotatoes: Cooked (raw, 5 by 2 in; about 2 1/2 per lb):																		
666	Baked in skin, peeled — 1 potato	114	64	160	2	1	—	—	—	37	46	66	1.0	342	9,230	.10	.08	.8	25
667	Boiled in skin, peeled — 1 potato	151	71	170	3	1	—	—	—	40	48	71	1.1	367	11,940	.14	.09	.9	26
668	Candied, 2 1/2 by 2-in piece — 1 piece	105	60	175	1	3	2.0	.8	.1	36	39	45	.9	200	6,620	.06	.04	.4	11
	Canned:																		
669	Solid pack (mashed) — 1 cup	255	72	275	5	1	—	—	—	63	64	105	2.0	510	19,890	.13	.10	1.5	36
670	Vacuum pack, piece 2 3/4 by 1 in — 1 piece	40	72	45	1	Trace	—	—	—	10	10	16	.3	80	3,120	.02	.02	.2	6
	Tomatoes:																		
671	Raw, 2 3/5-in diam. (3 per 12 oz pkg.) — 1 tomato	135	94	25	1	Trace	—	—	—	6	16	33	.6	300	1,110	.07	.05	.9	*28
672	Canned, solids and liquid — 1 cup	241	94	50	2	Trace	—	—	—	10	**14	46	1.2	523	2,170	.12	.07	1.7	41
673	Tomato catsup — 1 cup	273	69	290	5	1	—	—	—	69	60	137	2.2	991	3,820	.25	.19	4.4	41
674	Tomato catsup — 1 tbsp	15	69	15	Trace	Trace	—	—	—	4	3	8	.1	54	210	.01	.01	.2	2
	Tomato juice, canned:																		
675	Cup — 1 cup	243	94	45	2	Trace	—	—	—	10	17	44	2.2	552	1,940	.12	.07	1.9	39
676	Glass (6 fl oz) — 1 glass	182	94	35	2	Trace	—	—	—	8	13	33	1.6	413	1,460	.09	.05	1.5	29
677	Turnips, cooked, diced — 1 cup	155	94	35	1	Trace	—	—	—	8	54	37	.6	291	Trace	.06	.08	.5	34
	Turnip greens, cooked, drained:																		
678	From raw (leaves and stems) — 1 cup	145	94	30	3	Trace	—	—	—	5	252	49	1.5		8,270	.15	.33	.7	68
679	From frozen (chopped) — 1 cup	165	93	40	4	Trace	—	—	—	6	195	64	2.6	246	11,390	.08	.15	.7	31
680	Vegetables, mixed, frozen, cooked — 1 cup	182	83	115	6	1	—	—	—	24	46	115	2.4	348	9,010	.22	.13	2.0	15

MISCELLANEOUS ITEMS

(A)	(B)	(C)	(D)	(E)	(F)	(G)	(H)	(I)	(J)	(K)	(L)	(M)	(N)	(O)	(P)	(Q)	(R)	(S)
681	Baking powders for home use: Sodium aluminum sulfate: With monocalcium phosphate monohydrate	1 tsp	3.0	2	5	Trace	Trace	0	0	0	1	58	—	5	0	0	0	0	0
682	With monocalcium phosphate monohydrate, calcium sulfate	1 tsp	2.9	1	5	Trace	Trace	0	0	0	1	183	—	—	0	0	0	0	0
683	Straight phosphate	1 tsp	3.8	2	5	Trace	Trace	0	0	0	1	239	—	6	0	0	0	0	0
684	Low sodium	1 tsp	4.3	2	5	Trace	Trace	0	0	0	2	207	—	471	0	0	0	0	0
685	Barbecue sauce	1 cup	250	81	230	4	17	2.2	4.3	10.0	20	53	2.0	435	900	.03	.03	.8	13
686	Beverages, alcoholic: Gin, rum, vodka, whisky: 80-proof	1 1/2-fl oz jigger	42	67	95	—	0	0	0	0	Trace	—	—	1	—	—	—	—	—
687	90-proof	1 1/2-fl oz jigger	42	64	110	—	0	0	0	0	Trace	—	—	1	—	—	—	—	—
688	94-proof	1 1/2-fl oz jigger	42	62	116	—	0	0	0	0	Trace	—	—	1	—	—	—	—	—
689	100-proof	1 1/2-fl oz jigger	42	58	124	—	0	0	0	0	Trace	—	—	1	—	—	—	—	—
690	Wines: Dessert	3 1/2-fl oz glass	103	77	140	Trace	0	—	—	—	8	8	—	77	—	.01	.02	.2	—
691	Table	3 1/2-fl oz glass	102	86	85	Trace	0	—	—	—	4	9	—	94	—	.01	.01	.1	—
692	Beverages, carbonated, sweetened, nonalcoholic: Carbonated water	12 fl oz	366	92	115	0	0	0	0	0	29	—	—	—	0	0	0	0	0
693	Cola type	12 fl oz	369	90	145	0	0	0	0	0	37	—	—	—	0	0	0	0	0
694	Fruit-flavored sodas and Tom Collins mixer	12 fl oz	372	88	170	0	0	0	0	0	45	—	—	—	0	0	0	0	0
695	Ginger ale	12 fl oz	366	92	115	0	0	0	0	0	29	—	—	—	0	0	0	0	0
696	Root beer	12 fl oz	370	90	150	0	0	0	0	0	39	—	—	—	0	0	0	0	0
697	Chili powder. See Peppers, hot, red (item 642). Chocolate: Bitter or baking	1 oz	28	2	145	3	15	8.9	4.9	.4	8	22	1.9	235	20	.01	.07	.4	0
	Semisweet. See Candy, chocolate (item 539).																		
698	Gelatin, dry	1 7-g envelope	7	13	25	6	Trace	0	0	0	0	—	—	—	—	—	—	—	—
699	Gelatin dessert prepared with gelatin dessert powder and water	1 cup	240	84	140	4	0	0	0	0	34	—	—	—	—	—	—	—	—
700	Mustard, prepared, yellow	1 tsp or individual serving pouch or cup	5	80	5	Trace	Trace	—	—	—	Trace	4	.1	7	—	—	—	—	—
701	Olives, pickled, canned: Green	4 medium or 3 extra large or 2 giant	16[4]	78	15	Trace	2	.2	1.2	.1	Trace	8	.2	7	40	—	—	—	—
702	Ripe, Mission	3 small or 2 large	10[4]	73	15	Trace	2	.2	1.2	.2	Trace	9	.1	2	10	Trace	Trace	—	—
703	Pickles, cucumber: Dill, medium, whole, 3 3/4 in long, 1 1/4-in diam	1 pickle	65	93	5	Trace	Trace	—	—	—	1	17	.7	130	70	Trace	.01	Trace	4
704	Fresh-pack, slices 1 1/2-in diam, 1/4 in thick	2 slices	15	79	10	Trace	Trace	—	—	—	3	5	.3	—	20	Trace	Trace	Trace	1
705	Sweet, gherkin, small, whole, about 2 1/2 in long, 3/4-in diam	1 pickle	15	61	20	Trace	Trace	—	—	—	5	2	.2	—	10	Trace	Trace	Trace	1
706	Relish, finely chopped, sweet	1 tbsp	15	63	20	Trace	Trace	—	—	—	5	3	.1	—	—	—	—	—	—
	Popcorn. See items 476-478.																		
707	Popsicle, 3-fl oz size	1 popsicle	95	80	70	0	0	0	0	0	18	0	Trace	—	0	0	0	0	0

[1] Weight includes cores and stem ends. Without these parts, weight is 123 g.
[2] Based on year-round average. For tomatoes marketed from November through May, value is about 12 mg; from June through October, 32 mg.
[3] Applies to product without calcium salts added. Value for products with calcium salts added may be as much as 63 mg for whole tomatoes, 241 mg for cut forms.
[4] Weight includes pits. Without pits, weight is 13 g for item 701, 9 g for item 702.

MISCELLANEOUS ITEMS—Con.

(A)	(B)	(C)		(D)	(E)	(F)	(G)	(H)	(I)	(J)	(K)	(L)	(M)	(N)	(O)	(P)	(Q)	(R)	(S)
		Grams	Per cent	(cal)	Grams	Grams	Grams	Grams	Grams	Grams	Milligrams	Milligrams	Milligrams	Milligrams	International units	Milligrams	Milligrams	Milligrams	Milligrams
	Soups:																		
	Canned, condensed:																		
	Prepared with equal volume of milk:																		
708	Cream of chicken-----	245	85	180	7	10	4.2	3.6	1.3	15	172	152	.5	260	610	.05	.27	.7	2
709	Cream of mushroom----	245	83	215	7	14	5.4	2.9	4.6	16	191	169	.5	279	250	.05	.34	.7	1
710	Tomato--------------	250	84	175	7	7	3.4	1.7	1.0	23	168	155	.8	418	1,200	.10	.25	1.3	15
	Prepared with equal volume of water:																		
711	Bean with pork------	250	84	170	8	6	1.2	1.8	2.4	22	63	128	2.3	395	650	.13	.08	1.0	3
712	Beef broth, bouillon, consomme	240	96	30	5	0	0	0	0	3	Trace	31	.5	130	Trace	Trace	.02	1.2	—
713	Beef noodle---------	240	93	65	4	3	.6	.7	.8	7	7	48	1.0	77	50	.05	.07	1.0	Trace
714	Clam chowder, Manhattan type (with tomatoes, without milk)	245	92	80	2	3	.5	.4	1.3	12	34	47	1.0	184	880	.02	.02	1.0	—
715	Cream of chicken----	240	92	95	3	6	1.6	2.3	1.1	8	24	34	.5	79	410	.02	.05	.5	Trace
716	Cream of mushroom---	240	90	135	2	10	2.6	1.7	4.5	10	41	50	.5	98	70	.02	.12	.7	Trace
717	Minestrone----------	245	90	105	5	3	.7	.9	1.3	14	37	59	1.0	314	2,350	.07	.05	1.0	—
718	Split pea-----------	245	85	145	9	3	1.1	1.2	.4	21	29	149	1.5	270	440	.25	.15	1.5	1
719	Tomato--------------	245	91	90	2	3	.5	.5	1.0	16	15	34	.7	230	1,000	.05	.05	1.2	12
720	Vegetable beef------	245	92	80	5	2	—	—	—	10	12	49	.7	162	2,700	.05	.05	1.0	—
721	Vegetarian----------	245	92	80	2	2	—	—	—	13	20	39	1.0	172	2,940	.05	.05	1.0	—
	Dehydrated:																		
722	Bouillon cube, 1/2 in cube	4	4	5	1	Trace	—	—	—	Trace	—	—	—	4	—	—	—	—	—
	Mixes:																		
	Unprepared:																		
723	Onion--------------- 1 1/2-oz pkg	43	3	150	6	5	1.1	2.3	1.0	23	42	49	.6	238	30	.05	.03	.3	6
	Prepared with water:																		
724	Chicken noodle------	240	95	55	2	1	—	—	—	8	7	19	.2	19	50	.07	.05	.5	Trace
725	Onion---------------	240	96	35	1	1	—	—	—	6	10	12	.2	58	Trace	Trace	Trace	.5	2
726	Tomato-vegetable with noodles	240	93	65	1	1	—	—	—	12	7	19	.2	29	480	.05	.02	.5	5
727	Vinegar, cider------ 1 tbsp	15	94	Trace	0	0	—	—	—	1	1	1	.1	15	—	—	—	—	—
728	White sauce, medium, with enriched flour	250	73	405	10	31	19.3	7.8	.8	22	288	233	.5	348	1,150	.12	.43	.7	2
	Yeast:																		
729	Baker's, dry, active 1 pkg	7	5	20	3	Trace	—	—	—	3	3	90	1.1	140	Trace	.16	.38	2.6	Trace
730	Brewer's, dry------- 1 tbsp	8	5	25	3	Trace	—	—	—	3	[29]17	140	1.4	152	Trace	1.25	.34	3.0	Trace

[29]Value may vary from 6 to 60 mg.

APPENDIX G.

RECOMMENDED DAILY DIETARY ALLOWANCES (RDA)

(Designed for the maintenance of good nutrition of practically all healthy persons in the United States.)

Sex-age category	Age (Years From–To)	Weight Kilograms	Weight Pounds	Height Centimeters	Height Inches	Food energy Calories	Protein Grams	Calcium Milligrams	Phosphorus Milligrams	Iron Milligrams	Vitamin A International units	Thiamin Milligrams	Riboflavin Milligrams	Niacin Milligrams	Ascorbic acid Milligrams
Infants	0–0.5	6	14	60	24	kg x 117 / lb x 53.2	kg x 2.2 / lb x 1.0	360	240	10	1,400	0.3	0.4	5	35
	0.5–1	9	20	71	28	kg x 108 / lb x 49.1	kg x 2.0 / lb x 0.9	540	400	15	2,000	.5	.6	8	35
Children	1–3	13	28	86	34	1,300	23	800	800	15	2,000	.7	.8	9	40
	4–6	20	44	110	44	1,800	30	800	800	10	2,500	.9	1.1	12	40
	7–10	30	66	135	54	2,400	36	800	800	10	3,300	1.2	1.2	16	40
Males	11–14	44	97	158	63	2,800	44	1,200	1,200	18	5,000	1.4	1.5	18	45
	15–18	61	134	172	69	3,000	54	1,200	1,200	18	5,000	1.5	1.8	20	45
	19–22	67	147	172	69	3,000	54	800	800	10	5,000	1.5	1.8	20	45
	23–50	70	154	172	69	2,700	56	800	800	10	5,000	1.4	1.6	18	45
	51+	70	154	172	69	2,400	56	800	800	10	5,000	1.2	1.5	16	45
Females	11–14	44	97	155	62	2,400	44	1,200	1,200	18	4,000	1.2	1.3	16	45
	15–18	54	119	162	65	2,100	48	1,200	1,200	18	4,000	1.1	1.4	14	45
	19–22	58	128	162	65	2,100	46	800	800	18	4,000	1.1	1.4	14	45
	23–50	58	128	162	65	2,000	46	800	800	18	4,000	1.0	1.2	13	45
	51+	58	128	162	65	1,800	46	800	800	10	4,000	1.0	1.2	12	45
Pregnant						+300	+30	1,200	1,200	2+18	5,000	+ .3	+ .3	+2	60
Lactating						+500	+20	1,200	1,200	18	6,000	+ .3	+ .5	+4	80

APPENDIX H. CALORIC EXPENDITURE PER MINUTE FOR VARIOUS ACTIVITIES

Calorie Expenditure per Minute for Various Activities

Activity	90	99	108	117	125	134	143	152	161	170	178	187	196	205	213	222	231	240	249	257	266	275
Archery	3.1	3.4	3.7	4.0	4.5	4.6	4.9	5.2	5.5	5.8	6.1	6.4	6.7	7.0	7.3	7.6	7.9	8.2	8.5	8.8	9.1	9.4
Badminton (recreation)	3.4	3.8	4.1	4.4	4.8	5.1	5.4	5.6	6.1	6.4	6.8	7.1	7.4	7.8	8.1	8.3	8.8	9.1	9.4	9.8	10.1	10.4
Badminton (competition)	5.9	6.4	7.0	7.6	8.1	8.7	9.3	9.9	10.5	11.0	11.6	12.1	12.7	13.3	13.9	14.4	15.0	15.6	16.1	16.7	17.3	17.9
Baseball (player)	2.8	3.1	3.4	3.6	3.9	4.2	4.5	4.7	5.0	5.3	5.5	5.8	6.1	6.4	6.6	6.9	7.2	7.5	7.7	8.0	8.3	8.6
Baseball (pitcher)	3.5	3.9	4.3	4.6	5.0	5.3	5.7	6.0	6.4	6.7	7.1	7.4	7.8	8.1	8.5	8.8	9.2	9.5	9.9	10.2	10.6	10.9
Basketball (half-court)	2.5	3.3	3.5	3.8	4.1	4.4	4.7	4.9	5.3	5.6	5.9	6.2	6.4	6.7	7.0	7.3	7.5	7.6	8.2	8.5	8.8	9.0
Basketball (moderate)	4.2	4.6	5.0	5.5	5.9	6.3	6.7	7.1	7.5	7.9	8.3	8.8	9.2	9.6	10.0	10.4	10.9	11.1	11.6	12.1	12.5	12.9
Basketball (competition)	5.9	6.5	7.1	7.7	8.2	8.8	9.4	10.0	10.6	11.1	11.7	12.3	12.9	13.5	14.0	14.6	15.0	15.2	16.3	16.9	17.5	18.1
Bicycling (level) 5.5 mph	3.0	3.3	3.6	3.9	4.2	4.5	4.8	5.1	5.4	5.6	5.9	6.2	6.5	6.8	7.1	7.4	7.7	8.0	8.3	8.6	8.9	9.2
Bicycling (level) 13 mph	6.4	7.1	7.7	8.3	8.9	9.6	10.2	10.8	11.4	12.1	12.7	13.4	14.0	14.6	15.2	15.9	16.5	17.1	17.8	18.4	19.0	19.6
Bowling (nonstop)	4.0	4.4	4.8	5.2	5.6	5.9	6.3	6.7	7.1	7.5	7.9	8.3	8.7	9.1	9.5	9.8	10.2	10.6	11.0	11.4	11.8	12.2
Boxing (sparring)	3.0	3.3	3.6	3.9	4.2	4.5	4.8	5.1	5.4	5.6	5.9	6.2	6.5	6.8	7.1	7.4	7.7	8.0	8.3	8.6	8.9	9.2
Calisthenics	3.0	3.3	3.6	3.9	4.2	4.5	4.8	5.1	5.4	5.6	5.9	6.2	6.5	6.8	7.1	7.4	7.7	8.0	8.3	8.6	8.9	9.2
Canoeing, 2.5 mph	1.8	1.9	2.0	2.2	2.3	2.5	2.7	3.0	3.2	3.4	3.6	3.7	3.9	4.1	4.3	4.4	4.6	4.8	5.0	5.1	5.3	5.5
Canoeing, 4.0 mph	4.2	4.6	5.0	5.5	5.9	6.3	6.7	7.1	7.5	7.9	8.3	8.7	9.2	9.4	10.0	10.5	10.8	11.2	11.6	12.0	12.4	12.9
Dance, modern (moderate)	2.5	2.8	3.0	3.2	3.5	3.7	4.0	4.2	4.5	4.7	5.0	5.2	5.4	5.7	5.9	6.2	6.4	6.7	6.9	7.2	7.4	7.6
Dance, modern (vigorous)	3.4	3.7	4.1	4.4	4.7	5.1	5.4	5.7	6.1	6.4	6.7	7.1	7.4	7.7	8.1	8.4	8.7	9.1	9.4	9.7	10.1	10.4
Dance, fox-trot	2.7	2.9	3.2	3.4	3.7	4.0	4.2	4.5	4.7	5.0	5.3	5.5	5.8	6.0	6.3	6.6	6.8	7.1	7.3	7.6	7.9	8.1
Dance, rumba	4.2	4.6	5.0	5.4	5.8	6.2	6.6	7.0	7.4	7.8	8.2	8.6	9.0	9.4	9.8	10.2	10.6	11.0	11.5	11.9	12.3	12.6
Dance, square	4.1	4.5	4.9	5.3	5.7	6.1	6.5	6.9	7.3	7.8	8.1	8.5	8.9	9.3	9.7	10.1	10.5	10.9	11.3	11.7	12.1	12.4
Dance, waltz	3.1	3.4	3.7	4.0	4.3	4.6	4.9	5.2	5.5	5.8	6.1	6.4	6.7	7.0	7.3	7.6	7.9	8.2	8.5	8.8	9.1	9.4
Fencing (moderate)	3.0	3.3	3.6	3.9	4.2	4.5	4.8	5.1	5.4	5.6	6.0	6.2	6.5	6.8	7.1	7.4	7.7	8.0	8.3	8.6	8.9	9.2
Fencing (vigorous)	6.2	6.8	7.4	8.0	8.6	9.2	9.8	10.4	11.0	11.6	12.2	12.8	13.4	14.0	14.6	15.2	15.8	16.4	17.0	17.6	18.2	18.8
Football (moderate)	3.0	3.3	3.6	4.0	4.2	4.5	4.8	5.1	5.4	5.7	6.0	6.2	6.5	6.8	7.1	7.4	7.7	8.0	8.3	8.6	8.9	9.2
Football (vigorous)	5.0	5.5	6.0	6.4	6.9	7.4	7.9	8.4	8.9	9.4	9.8	10.3	10.8	11.3	11.8	12.3	12.8	13.2	13.7	14.2	14.7	15.2
Golf, 2-some	3.3	3.6	3.9	4.2	4.5	4.8	5.2	5.5	5.8	6.1	6.4	6.7	7.1	7.4	7.7	8.0	8.3	8.6	9.0	9.3	9.6	10.0
Golf, 4-some	2.4	2.7	2.9	3.2	3.4	3.6	3.9	4.1	4.3	4.6	4.8	5.1	5.3	5.5	5.8	6.0	6.2	6.5	6.7	7.0	7.2	7.4
Handball	5.9	6.4	7.0	7.6	8.1	8.7	9.3	9.9	10.4	11.0	11.6	12.1	12.7	13.3	13.9	14.4	15.0	15.6	16.1	16.7	17.3	17.9
Hiking, 40 lb. pack, 3.0 mph	4.1	4.5	4.9	5.3	5.7	6.1	6.5	6.9	7.3	7.7	8.1	8.5	8.9	9.3	9.7	10.1	10.5	10.9	11.3	11.7	12.1	12.5
Horseback Riding (walk)	2.0	2.3	2.4	2.6	2.8	3.0	3.1	3.3	3.5	3.7	3.9	4.1	4.3	4.5	4.7	4.9	5.1	5.3	5.5	5.7	5.8	6.0
Horseback Riding (trot)	4.1	4.4	4.8	5.2	5.6	6.0	6.4	6.8	7.1	7.6	8.0	8.4	8.8	9.3	9.6	10.0	10.4	10.8	11.2	11.6	12.0	12.4
Horseshoe Pitching	2.1	2.3	2.5	2.7	3.0	3.3	3.4	3.6	3.8	4.0	4.2	4.4	4.6	4.8	5.0	5.2	5.4	5.6	5.8	6.0	6.3	6.5
Judo, Karate	7.7	8.5	9.2	10.0	10.7	11.5	12.2	13.0	13.7	14.5	15.2	16.0	16.7	17.5	18.2	19.0	19.7	20.5	21.2	22.0	22.7	23.5
Mountain Climbing	6.0	6.5	7.2	7.8	8.4	9.0	9.6	10.1	10.7	11.3	11.9	12.5	13.1	13.7	14.3	14.8	15.4	16.0	16.6	17.2	17.8	18.4
Paddleball, Racquetball	5.9	6.4	7.0	7.6	8.1	8.7	9.3	9.9	10.4	11.0	11.6	12.1	12.7	13.3	13.9	14.4	15.0	15.6	16.1	16.7	17.3	17.9
Pool, Billiards	1.1	1.2	1.3	1.4	1.5	1.6	1.7	1.8	1.9	2.0	2.1	2.2	2.4	2.5	2.6	2.7	2.8	2.9	3.0	3.1	3.2	3.3
Push Ups	4.3	4.7	5.1	5.6	6.0	6.4	6.8	7.2	7.7	8.1	8.5	8.9	9.4	9.8	10.2	10.6	11.0	11.5	11.9	12.3	12.7	13.2
Racquetball	6.0	6.6	7.2	7.8	8.3	8.9	9.5	10.1	10.7	11.3	11.9	12.5	13.1	13.7	14.2	14.8	15.4	16.0	16.6	17.2	17.8	18.4

Body Weight

Calorie Expenditure per Minute for Various Activities

Activity	Body Weight 90	99	108	117	125	134	143	152	161	170	178	187	196	205	213	222	231	240	249	257	266	275
Rowing (recreation)	3.0	3.3	3.6	3.9	4.2	4.5	4.8	5.1	5.4	5.6	6.0	6.2	6.5	6.8	7.1	7.5	7.7	8.0	8.3	8.6	8.9	9.2
Rowing (machine)	8.2	9.0	9.8	10.6	11.4	12.2	13.0	13.8	14.6	15.4	16.2	17.0	17.8	18.6	19.4	20.2	21.0	21.8	22.6	23.4	24.2	25.0
Running, 11-min. mile 5.5 mph	6.4	7.1	7.7	8.3	9.0	9.6	10.2	10.8	11.5	12.1	12.7	13.4	14.0	14.6	15.2	15.9	16.5	17.1	17.8	18.4	19.0	19.6
Running, 8.5-min. mile 7 mph	8.4	9.2	10.0	10.8	11.7	12.5	13.3	14.1	14.9	15.7	16.6	17.4	18.2	19.0	19.8	20.7	21.5	22.3	23.1	23.9	24.8	25.6
Running, 7-min. mile 9 mph	9.3	10.2	11.1	12.0	12.9	13.9	14.8	15.7	16.6	17.5	18.4	19.3	20.2	21.1	22.1	23.0	23.9	24.8	25.7	26.6	27.5	28.4
Running, 5-min. mile 12 mph	11.8	13.0	14.1	15.3	16.4	17.6	18.7	19.9	21.0	22.2	23.3	24.5	25.6	26.8	27.9	29.1	30.2	31.4	32.5	33.7	34.9	36.0
Sailing	1.8	2.0	2.1	2.3	2.4	2.7	2.8	3.0	3.2	3.4	3.6	3.8	3.9	4.1	4.3	4.4	4.6	4.8	5.0	5.1	5.3	5.5
Sit ups	4.3	4.7	5.1	5.6	6.0	6.4	6.8	7.2	7.7	8.1	8.5	8.9	9.4	9.8	10.2	10.6	11.0	11.5	11.9	12.3	12.7	13.2
Sprinting	13.8	15.2	16.6	17.9	19.2	20.5	21.9	23.3	24.7	26.1	27.3	28.7	30.0	31.4	32.7	34.0	35.4	36.8	38.1	39.4	40.7	42.2
Skating (moderate)	3.4	3.8	4.1	4.4	4.8	5.1	5.4	5.8	6.1	6.4	6.8	7.1	7.4	7.8	8.1	8.3	8.8	9.1	9.4	9.8	10.1	10.4
Skating (vigorous)	6.2	6.8	7.4	8.0	8.6	9.2	9.8	10.4	11.0	11.6	12.2	12.8	13.4	14.0	14.6	15.2	15.8	16.4	17.0	17.6	18.2	18.8
Skiing (downhill)	5.8	6.4	6.9	7.5	8.1	8.6	9.2	9.8	10.3	10.9	11.4	12.0	12.6	13.1	13.7	14.3	14.8	15.4	16.0	16.5	17.1	17.7
Skiing (level, 5 mph)	7.0	7.7	8.4	9.1	9.8	10.5	11.1	11.8	12.5	13.2	13.9	14.6	15.2	15.9	16.6	17.3	18.0	18.7	19.4	20.0	20.7	21.4
Skiing (racing downhill)	9.9	10.9	11.9	12.9	13.7	14.7	15.7	16.7	17.7	18.7	19.6	20.6	21.6	22.6	23.4	24.4	25.4	26.4	27.4	28.3	29.3	30.2
Snowshoeing (2.3 mph)	3.7	4.1	4.5	4.8	5.2	5.5	5.9	6.3	6.7	7.0	7.4	7.8	8.1	8.5	8.8	9.2	9.6	9.9	10.3	10.6	11.0	11.4
Snowshoeing (2.5 mph)	5.4	5.9	6.5	7.0	7.5	8.0	8.6	9.1	9.7	10.2	10.7	11.2	11.8	12.3	12.8	13.3	13.9	14.4	14.9	15.4	16.0	16.5
Soccer	5.4	5.9	6.4	6.9	7.5	8.0	8.5	9.0	9.6	10.1	10.6	11.1	11.6	12.2	12.7	13.2	13.7	14.3	14.8	15.3	15.8	16.9
Squash	6.2	6.8	7.5	8.1	8.7	9.3	9.9	10.5	11.1	11.7	12.3	12.9	13.5	14.2	14.8	15.4	16.0	16.6	17.2	17.8	18.4	19.0
Stationary Running, 140 counts/min.	14.6	16.1	17.5	18.9	20.4	21.8	23.2	24.6	26.1	27.5	28.9	30.4	31.8	33.2	34.6	36.1	37.5	38.9	40.4	41.8	43.2	44.6
Swimming, pleasure 25 yds./min.	3.6	4.0	4.3	4.7	5.0	5.4	5.7	6.1	6.4	6.8	7.1	7.5	7.8	8.2	8.5	8.9	9.2	9.6	10.0	10.3	10.6	11.0
Swimming, back 20 yds./min.	2.3	2.6	2.8	3.0	3.2	3.5	3.7	3.9	4.1	4.2	4.6	4.8	5.0	5.3	5.5	5.7	6.0	6.2	6.4	6.6	6.9	7.1
Swimming, back 30 yds./min.	3.2	3.5	3.8	4.1	4.4	4.7	5.1	5.4	5.7	6.0	6.3	6.6	6.9	7.2	7.4	7.9	8.2	8.5	8.8	9.1	9.4	9.7
Swimming, back 40 yds./min.	5.0	5.5	5.8	6.5	7.0	7.5	7.9	8.5	8.9	9.4	9.9	10.4	10.9	11.4	11.9	12.3	12.8	13.3	13.8	14.3	14.8	15.3
Swimming, breast 20 yds./min.	2.9	3.2	3.4	3.8	4.0	4.3	4.6	4.9	5.1	5.4	5.7	6.0	6.3	6.5	6.8	7.1	7.4	7.7	7.9	8.2	8.5	8.8
Swimming, breast 30 yds./min.	4.3	4.8	5.2	5.7	6.0	6.4	6.9	7.3	7.7	8.1	8.6	9.0	9.4	9.9	10.3	10.8	11.1	11.5	11.9	12.4	13.0	13.3
Swimming, breast 40 yds./min.	5.8	6.3	6.9	7.5	8.0	8.6	9.2	9.7	10.3	10.8	11.4	12.0	12.5	13.1	13.7	14.2	14.8	15.4	15.9	16.5	17.0	17.6

Calorie Expenditure per Minute for Various Activities

	Body Weight																					
	90	99	108	117	125	134	143	152	161	170	178	187	196	205	213	222	231	240	249	257	266	275
Swimming, butterfly 50 yds./min.	7.0	7.7	8.4	9.1	9.8	10.5	11.1	11.9	12.5	13.2	13.9	14.6	15.2	15.9	16.6	17.3	18.0	18.7	19.4	20.0	20.7	21.4
Swimming, crawl 20 yds./min.	2.9	3.2	3.4	3.8	4.0	4.3	4.6	4.9	5.1	5.4	5.7	5.8	6.3	6.5	6.8	7.1	7.3	7.7	7.9	8.2	8.5	8.8
Swimming, crawl 45 yds./min.	5.2	5.8	6.3	6.8	7.3	7.8	8.3	8.8	9.3	9.8	10.4	10.9	11.4	11.9	12.4	12.9	13.4	13.9	14.4	15.0	15.5	16.0
Swimming, crawl 50 yds./min.	6.4	7.0	7.6	8.3	8.9	9.5	10.1	10.7	11.4	12.0	12.6	13.2	13.9	14.5	15.1	15.7	16.3	17.0	17.4	17.9	18.8	19.5
Table Tennis	2.3	2.6	2.8	3.0	3.2	3.5	3.7	3.9	4.1	4.2	4.6	4.8	5.0	5.3	5.5	5.7	6.0	6.2	6.4	6.6	6.9	7.1
Tennis (recreation)	4.2	4.6	5.0	5.4	5.8	6.2	6.6	7.0	7.4	7.8	8.2	8.6	9.0	9.4	9.8	10.2	10.6	11.0	11.5	11.9	12.3	12.6
Tennis (competition)	5.9	6.4	7.0	7.6	8.1	8.7	9.3	9.9	10.4	11.0	11.6	12.1	12.7	13.3	13.9	14.4	15.0	15.6	16.1	16.7	17.3	17.9
Timed Calisthenics	8.8	9.6	10.5	11.4	12.2	13.1	13.9	14.8	15.6	16.5	17.4	18.2	19.1	19.9	20.8	21.5	22.5	23.9	24.2	25.1	25.9	26.8
Volleyball (moderate)	3.4	3.8	4.0	4.4	4.8	5.1	5.4	5.8	6.1	6.4	6.8	7.1	7.4	7.8	8.1	8.3	8.8	9.1	9.4	9.8	10.1	10.4
Volleyball (vigorous)	5.9	6.4	7.0	7.6	8.1	8.7	9.3	9.9	10.4	11.0	11.6	12.1	12.7	13.3	13.9	14.4	15.0	15.6	16.1	16.7	17.3	17.9
Walking (2.0 mph)	2.1	2.3	2.5	2.7	2.9	3.1	3.3	3.5	3.7	4.0	4.2	4.4	4.6	4.8	5.0	5.2	5.4	5.6	5.8	6.0	6.2	6.4
Walking (4.5 mph)	4.0	4.4	4.7	5.1	5.5	5.9	6.3	6.7	7.1	7.5	7.8	8.2	8.6	9.0	9.4	9.8	10.1	10.6	10.9	11.3	11.7	12.0
Walking 110-120 steps/min.	3.1	3.4	3.7	4.0	4.3	4.7	5.0	5.3	5.6	5.9	6.2	6.5	6.8	7.1	7.4	7.7	8.0	8.3	8.6	8.9	9.2	9.5
Waterskiing	4.7	5.1	5.6	6.1	6.5	7.0	7.4	7.9	8.3	8.8	9.3	9.7	10.2	10.6	11.1	11.5	12.0	12.5	12.9	13.4	13.8	14.3
Weight Training	4.7	5.1	5.7	6.2	6.7	7.0	7.5	7.9	8.4	8.9	9.4	9.9	10.3	10.8	11.1	11.7	12.2	12.6	13.1	13.5	14.0	14.4
Wrestling	7.7	8.5	9.2	10.0	10.7	11.5	12.2	13.0	13.7	14.5	15.2	16.0	16.7	17.5	18.2	19.0	19.7	20.5	21.2	22.0	22.7	23.5

From Consolazio, Johnson and Pecora, *Physiological Measurements of Metabolic Functions in Man*, McGraw-Hill, 1963.

GOING BEYOND
Lab Reports

LAB 1
STUDENT CONSENT FORM

As a student in this exercise course you will be involved in several exercise conditioning and testing programs. A series of tests has been designed to determine the status of various personal health factors. All results will be used as base data to establish training programs related to modification and improvement of your fitness, muscle tone and body proportions.

The activities which will be used to reach the student's objectives as determined by pretests include:

1. jog and walk
2. jump rope activity
3. isometrics
4. weight training
5. correctives for posture
6. progressive relaxation
7. circuit training
8. aquadynamics
9. aerobic dance
10. resistance weight training
11. additional selections

In signing this consent form you state that you have read and understand the nature of these activities. You furthermore state that you are entering into these activities of your own free will and that you may withdraw from participation at any time. Assuredly, every effort will be made to insure your safe participation in this class. All activity will be performed within your personal limitations and capabilities.

Please indicate any medical related problems or other conditions that need to be considered in developing a personal health program for you.

Name of Family Physician _____

Name of Applicant (print) _____

Signature of Applicant _____

Address _____

Phone _____

Student Number _____

Indicate medical limitations _____

_____

_____

LAB 2
PRE-EXERCISE MEDICAL HISTORY FORM

NAME _____ AGE _____ DATE _____

ADDRESS _____ PHONE _____

OCCUPATION _____ HT _____ WT _____

DOCTOR'S NAME _____ PHONE _____

Past History   (Mark X if Yes)

(Have you ever had?)
Dates

Diabetes ( ) _____
Rheumatic Fever ( ) _____
Heart Murmur ( ) _____
High Blood Pressure ( ) _____
Any Heart Trouble ( ) _____
Disease of Arteries ( ) _____
Varicose Veins ( ) _____
Lung Disease ( ) _____
Operations ( ) _____
Epilepsy ( ) _____
Cancer ( ) _____
Anemia ( ) _____
Injuries to Back, Knees, ( ) _____
  Ankles, etc.
Explain:

Family History (Have any of your relatives had?)

Age   **Relative**

Heart Attacks ( ) _____ _____
High Blood Pressure ( ) _____ _____
High Cholesterol Levels ( ) _____ _____
Diabetes ( ) _____ _____
Congenital Heart Diseases ( ) _____ _____
Heart Operations ( ) _____ _____
Cancer ( ) _____ _____
Stroke ( ) _____ _____
Other: ( ) _____ _____
Explain:

Present Symptoms Review

(Have you recently had?)   **Date**

Chest Pain ( ) _____
Shortness of Breath ( ) _____
Heart Palpitations ( ) _____
Cough on Exertion ( ) _____

Explain:

Date

Coughing of Blood ( ) _____
Back Pain ( ) _____
Swollen, Stiff or Painful Joints ( ) _____

LAB 2, CONTINUED

Risk Factors

1. **Smoking**   Yes   No

   Cigarettes ( ) ( )   How many?_____ How many years?_____

   Cigar   ( ) ( )   How many?_____ How many years?_____

   Pipe   ( ) ( )   How many times a day?_____ How many years?_____

   How old were you when you started?_____

   In case you have stopped, when did you?_____

   Why?_____

2. **Diet**

   What is your weight now?_____ 1 year ago?_____ At age 21?_____

   Are you dieting?_____ Why?_____

3. **Exercise**

   Do you engage in any exercise, fitness, or recreational activities?_____

   What?_____ How often?_____

   How far do you think you walk each day?_____

   Is your occupation:

Sedentary	( )	Active	( )
Inactive	( )	Heavy Work	( )

   Do you have discomfort, shortness of breath, or pain with moderate exercise?_____

   Were you a high school or college athlete?_____ Specify_____

Mark any of the medicines you are now taking

   _____ Mood elevators (pills for depression)

   _____ Pep or diet pills (like dexadrine)

   _____ Tranquilizers, sedatives, nerve or sleeping pills (Miltown, Librium, Phenobarbital, Nembutal, Seconal, etc.)

   _____ Pain pills (Demerol, Codeine, Morphine, etc.)

   _____ Antihistamines or allergy pills

   _____ Blood pressure pills

LAB 3
FITNESS PROFILE CHART

NAME_____ SECTION_____ DATE _____

FITNESS TEST	Initial Score	Rating	Final Score	Rating	Change
CARDIOVASCULAR					
Resting Heart Rate					
Walking Test					
Sit/Stand Test					
12 Min. Run/1.5 Mile Run					
FLEXIBILITY					
Bend and Reach					
Shoulder Lift					
Trunk Extension					
MUSCULAR ENDURANCE					
Sit-Ups					
Push-Ups					
Static Push-Up					

LAB 3, CONTINUED

Conclusions:

Initial Tests

What do the initial tests indicate as your area of greatest weakness?

Area of greatest strength?

Final Tests

1. In which areas did you show significant improvement?

2. What were the reasons for your areas of improvement?

3. If you did not improve on any of the tests what do you think is the reason?

4. What implications do your results have for the future?

LAB 4
CONTRACT FOR CHANGE

NAME _____SECTION _____DATE _____

Establishing goals for change is an important process. Individuals must determine the changes they desire and make a plan as to how best achieve these changes. By your commitment this endeavor could bring about lifestyle changes.

Procedure:

Indicate the goals that you currently desire to achieve during the next semester. Be specific within each general area.

Goal	Steps to Reach the Goal

1. **Fitness**

   A.   Cardiovascular Endurance

   B.   Flexibility

   C.   Muscular Endurance

2. **Body Composition**

   A.   Weight

   B.   Body Fat Percentage

3. **Body Measurements**

4. **Posture**

LAB 4, CONTINUED

Conclusions

1. Which goals do you feel will be the most difficult for you to achieve?

2. What type of assistance do you need to help you achieve these goals?

3. Do you feel you are well motivated to achieve these goals?

LAB 5
GOAL ASSESSMENT

NAME _____ SECTION _____ DATE _____

The purpose of this lab is to compare your projected goals to those you actually experienced in your exercise program. Before starting your fitness routine, circle the appropriate responses to the list of reasons why most people exercise.

If the statement reflects a major goal, circle 2.
If the statement reflects a minor goal, circle 1.

		Before		After	
1.	To promote strong healthy bones	2	1	2	1
2.	To control the physical and emotional stress in daily living	2	1	2	1
3.	To increase productivity	2	1	2	1
4.	To lose or maintain desirable weight	2	1	2	1
5.	To reduce the chances of contracting cardiovascular disease	2	1	2	1
6.	To socialize and have fun	2	1	2	1
7.	To sleep better	2	1	2	1
8.	To develop an attractive body	2	1	2	1
9.	To improve blood chemistry	2	1	2	1
10.	To improve self-esteem	2	1	2	1

LAB 5, CONTINUED

11. To increase energy level   2   1   2   1

12. To develop muscular strength   2   1   2   1

13. To develop muscular endurance   2   1   2   1

14. To increase flexibility   2   1   2   1

15. To learn about weight management 2   1   2   1

16. To improve sex life   2   1   2   1

17. To improve cardiovascular endurance 2   1   2   1

18. To improve posture   2   1   2   1

19. To increase resistance to disease   2   1   2   1

20. To improve coordination   2   1   2   1

1. Add the circled numbers in column A and divide by 20 to get your average score.

2. Repeat the procedure for column B.

3. Which column has the highest number?

4. Were there more or fewer benefits derived from your aerobic exercise experience?

5. Explain.

LAB 6

ANALYSIS OF BODY FAT PERCENTAGES

NAME _____ SECTION_____ DATE_____

Determination of the percentage of body fat can be made by measurement with a skinfold caliper. A pinch of skin is pulled away from the underlying muscle and the thickness of the fold is measured with the caliper.

Results: Skinfold Measurements

FEMALES

Triceps (arm)_____

Abdomen _____

Hip (Ilium)_____

TOTAL _____

MALES

Chest_____

Hip (Ilium)_____

Abdomen _____

Side (Axilla)_____

TOTAL _____

Percentage of Body Fat: (See Appendix A)

Sum of all Scores =_____

Rating of Individual Measurements

FEMALES

Triceps _____

Abdomen_____

Hip (Ilium)_____

TOTAL _____

MALES

Chest_____

Hip (Ilium)_____

Abdomen _____

Side (Axilla)_____

TOTAL _____

Average of Scores = _____

Rating   = _____

LAB 6, CONTINUED

Conclusions:

1. How does your percentage of body fat compare with the optimal percentage (15 % for males, 20 % for females)?

2. What implications do these results have for improvement of your body composition?

LAB 7
ANALYSIS OF BODY COMPOSITION

NAME_____ SECTION_____ DATE_____

Age_____Height_____Target Weight_____

Initial **Body Weight**_____Final Body Weight_____Change_____

Initial **Body Fat %**_____Final Body Fat %_____Change_____

GIRTH MEASUREMENTS

Site	Initial Score	Desirable Score	Final Score	Actual Change
Chest (Bust)				
Waist				
Abdomen				
Hips				
Thigh: right				
left				
Calf: right				
left				
Ankle: right				
left				
Upper arm: right				
left				
Wrist				

LAB 7, CONTINUED

Conclusions:

Initial Tests

What do the initial tests indicate as your areas of greatest concern?

Final Tests

1. In which areas did you show significant improvement?

2. Which areas do you feel still need improvement?

3. What implications do your results have for the future?

LAB 8
NUTRITION AND DIET ANALYSIS

NAME_____ SECTION_____ DATE_____

Procedure:

1. Record everything you eat or drink for five days on the chart pro-vided. Record what was consumed, how much, and the time of day. Eat as normally as you can.

2. Using Appendix F, estimate the number of calories, grams of carbo-hydrates, protein, fat, and intake of the designated vitamins and minerals, or follow your instructor's directions for using the com-puterized diet analysis program.

Analysis:

1. Total all columns for each day and for the five day period.
2. Total all calories for each meal for each day.
3. Transfer figures to Diet Recall Summary Form.
4. Determine the average daily intake in all columns by dividing by 5.
5. Determine the average calories from fat, protein, and carbohydrate by multiplying the daily average by 9, 4, and 4, respectively.
6. Determine the percent of carbohydrate, fat, and protein intake by di-viding total calories into daily average in area and compare with optimal.
7. Compare your intake of vitamins and minerals with the RDA.

Conclusions:

1. On how many days out of the five did you eat properly from the four basic food groups?

2. Which group do you tend to omit?

3. In which group do you tend to overeat?

LAB 8, CONTINUED

4. How did your percentage of proteins, carbohydrates and fats compare with the optimal amount recommended?

5. What was the highest calorie food per serving that you ate or drank?

6. Which food gave you the highest amount of saturated fat?

7. When do you tend to eat the most calories?

8. What empty calories (no nutritional value) did you consume?

9. Do you snack? How much? What?

10. Could you include more healthful snacks? What?

11. Do you drink enough fluids daily?

12. On the basis of this analysis, what specific recommendations do you have regarding your current eating habits (foods you need to eliminate or cut back on, foods you need to eat more, low-calorie snacks you could select, etc.)

NAME_____SECTION_____DATE_____

Day	Time	Food	Amount	Calories	Protein Grams	Fat	Saturated Fat	Unsaturated Fat	Carbohydrates	Calcium	Phosphorus	Iron	Potassium	Vitamin A	Thiamin	Riboflavin	Niacin	Vitamin C

Day	Time	Food	Amount	Calories	Protein Grams	Fat	Saturated Fat	Unsaturated Fat	Carbohydrates	Calcium	Phosphorus	Iron	Potassium	Vitamin A	Thiamin	Riboflavin	Niacin	Vitamin C

LABORATORY 8, *CONTINUED*

NAME_____SECTION_____DATE_____

1. Calorie Analysis (Totals for each meal)

Days	1	2	3	4	5	6	7	8	9	10
Breakfast										
Lunch										
Dinner										
Snacks										
TOTALS										

2. Total Nutrients for 5 Days

A. Total calories_____

B. Total grams of protein_____

C. Total grams of fat_____

D. Total grams of saturated fat_____

E. Total grams of unsaturated fat_____

F. Total grams of carbohydrates_____

3. Average Nutrients per Day (Divide above by 5)

A. Average calories_____

B. Average grams of protein_____

C. Average grams of fat_____

D. Average grams of saturated fat_____

E. Average grams of unsaturated fat_____

F. Average grams of carbohydrates_____

4. **Average Calories Per Day Per Nutrient**

    A. Multiply average grams of protein per day by 4

    B. Multiply average grams of fat by 9

    C. Multiply average grams of saturated fat by 9

    D. Multiply average grams of unsaturated fat by 9

    E. Multiply average grams of carbohydrates by 4

5. **Percentage of Calories from Each Nutrient**

    A. Divide average calories per day from protein by average total calories per day.

    Total calories per day _____) Calories from protein

    B. Divide average calories per day from fat by average total calories per day.

    Total calories per day _____) Calories from fat

    C. Divide average calories per day from unsaturated fat by average total calories per day.

    Total calories per day _____) Calories from unsaturated fat

    D. Divide average calories per day from saturated fat by average total calories per day.

    Total calories per day _____) Calories from saturated fat

    E. Divide average calories per day from carbohydrates by average total calories per day.

    Total calories per day _____) Calories from carbohydrates

LAB 9
WEIGHT CONTROL CONTRACT

NAME_____ SECTION_____ DATE_____

Calorie Expenditure

1. Exercise Preference_____

2. Calories extended per minute (see Appendix H)_____

3. Number of minutes to exercise each day_____

4. Calories expended per day (line 2 × line 3)_____

Calorie Intake

5. Average caloric intake (from Lab 8 — Nutrition and Diet)_____

6. Calorie reduction per day to lose 2 pounds per week

   − 1,000 _____

7. Total daily calorie intake, without exercise 2 pounds a week

   (line 5 − line 6) _____

8. Daily calorie intake to lose 2 pounds per week, including exercise

   (line 7 + line 4)_____

   (*Note:* This total should not be below 1200 calories for women or 1500 calories for men.)

Contract Agreement

Height _____ Present weight _____ Target weight _____

My goal is to lose (gain) _____ pounds in _____ weeks. _____

_____	_____	_____
Signature	Date	Approval
_____	_____	_____
Contract Completion Date	Weight	Actual Change

WEEKLY WEIGHT RECORD

Weeks

Weight change in pounds	1	2	3	4	5	6	7	8	9	10	11	12	13	14	15	16
1																
2																
3																
4																
5																
6																
7																
8																
9																
10																
11																
12																
13																
14																
15																
16																
17																
18																
19																
20																

LAB 10

TARGET HEART RATE ZONE

NAME_____ SECTION_____ DATE_____

Target heart rate zone identifies for each person the safe and comfortable area in which cardiovascular exercise should occur to achieve a training effect.

Procedure

1. First, you must determine your maximum heart rate according to your age.

   The formula is: 220 − Age = Maximum Heart Rate.

   Example: 220
   <u>− 19</u>
   201 MHR

   It is not safe for you to work at a rate this high. Therefore, we must identify your TARGET HEART RATE ZONE, the safe upper limit and minimum lower limit necessary for cardiovascular improvement to occur.

2. It is important to consider your current resting heart rate because that is your individual starting point during exercise.

   201 (MHR) − Resting Heart Rate = Heart Rate Reserve

   Example: 201 (MHR)
   <u>− 68</u> (RHR)
   133 Heart Rate Reserve

3. The lower limit for a training effect is 70%:

   133 (Heart Rate Reserve) × .70 + RHR = Target Zone Lower Limit

   Example: 133
   .70
   93.10
   <u>+ 68</u>   RHR
   161.10 = Target Zone Lower Limit

4. The safe upper limit is 85%:

   133 (Heart Rate Reserve) × .85 + RHR = Target Zone Upper Limit

   Example: 133
   .85
   113.05
   <u>+ 68.00</u> RHR
   181.05 Target Zone Upper Limit

Assignment: Using the formula described above, compute your target heart rate for the 70% and 85% limits, using the form provided on the next page.

LAB 10, CONTINUED

Lower Limit	*Upper Limit*
220	220
_____	_____
_____	_____
_____	_____
_____	_____
____.70____	____.85____
_____	_____
_____	_____
_____	_____

Conclusions:

1. What is your 10 second pulse count for your lower limit?_____
   For your upper limit?_____

2. What should you do if you find that you are not reaching your lower limit?

3. What should you do if you find that you are exceeding your upper limit?

LAB 11
EXERCISE RECORDING FORM

NAME_____ SECTION_____ DATE_____

Target Heart Rate: Lower Limit_____Upper Limit_____

| DATE | FITNESS AREA | TYPE OF EXERCISE | ACTUAL WORKOUT TIME | HEART RATE | | | CALORIES BURNED |
				PRE EX.	POST EX.	FIVE MIN.	

LAB 12
BLOOD PRESSURE RECORD

NAME_____ SECTION_____ DATE_____

Blood pressure is a record of the pressure generated by the outflow of blood against the arterial walls. The highest reading is the **systolic** and represents peak pressure in your arteries during the contraction phase of the heart. The lowest pressure in the arteries is the **diastolic** and represents the pressure during the relaxation phase. The acceptable range for your blood pressure is stated as

SYSTOLIC = 120 $\pm$ 20 or 100 – 140

DIASTOLIC = 80 $\pm$ 10 or 70 – 90

Assignment:

Secure a record of your blood pressure for five days from any reliable source: doctor, nurse, school nurse, athletic trainer, home blood pressure unit, school fitness lab, etc.

Results:

	DATE	TIME	BLOOD PRESSURE READING	WHERE CHECKED
1.				
2.				
3.				
4.				
5.				

Conclusions:

1. What is your typical blood pressure?

2. Does your blood pressure level indicate you are at a safe level?

3. What might cause fluctuations or variations in one's blood pressure?

LAB 13 — Heart Attack Risk Factors

NAME_____ SECTION_____ DATE_____

The purpose of this game is to give you an estimate of your chances of suffering heart attack. The game is played by marking squares which — from left to right — represent an increase in your *risk factors.* These are medical conditions and habits associated with an increased danger of heart attack. Not all risk factors are measurable enough to be included in this game.

Rules:

Study each risk factor and its row. Find the box applicable to you and circle the large number in it. For example, if you are 37, circle the number in the box labeled 31-40.

After checking out all the rows, add the circled numbers. This total — your score — is an estimate of your risk.

If You Score:

6-11 — Risk well below average

12-17 — Risk below average

18-24 — Risk generally average

25-31 — Risk moderate

32-40 — Risk at a dangerous level

41-62 — Danger urgent. See your doctor now.

Heredity:

Count parents, grandparents, brothers, and sisters who have had heart attack and/or stroke.

Tobacco Smoking:

If you inhale deeply and smoke a cigarette way down, add one to your classification. Do *not* subtract because you think you do not inhale or smoke only a half inch on a cigarette.

Exercise:

Lower your score one point if you exercise regularly and frequently.

Cholesterol or Saturated Fat Intake Level:

A cholesterol blood test is best. If you can't get one from your doctor, then estimate honestly the percentage of solid fats you eat. These are usually of animal origin — lard, cream, butter, and beef and lamb fat. If you eat much of this, your cholesterol level probably will be high. The United States average, 40 percent, is too high for good health.

Blood Pressure:

If you have no recent reading but have passed an insurance or industrial examination chances are you are 140 or less.

Sex:

This line takes into account the fact that men have from 6 to 10 times more heart attacks than women of child bearing age.

AGE	10 to 20	21 to 30	31 to 40	41 to 50	51 to 60	61 to 70
HEREDITY	No known history of heart disease	1 relative with cardiovascular disease Over 60	2 relatives with cardiovascular disease Over 60	1 relative with cardiovascular disease Under 60	2 relatives with cardiovascular disease Under 60	3 relatives with cardiovascular disease Under 60
WEIGHT	More than 5 lbs. below standard weight	−5 to + 5 lbs standard weight	6-20 lbs over weight	21-35 lbs over weight	36-50 lbs over weight	51-65 lbs over weight
TOBACCO SMOKING	Non-user	Cigar and/or pipe	10 cigarettes or less a day	20 cigarettes a day	30 cigarettes a day	40 cigarettes a day or more
EXERCISE	Intensive occupational and recreational exertion	Moderate occupational and recreational exertion	Sedentary work and intense recreational exertion	Sedentary occupational and moderate exertion	Sedentary work and light recreational	Complete lack of all exercise
CHOLES-TEROL OR FAT % IN DIET	Cholesterol below 180 mg % Diet contains no animal or solid fats	Cholesterol 181-205 mg % Diet contains 10% animal or solid fats	Cholesterol 206-230 mg % Diet contains 20% animal or solid fats	Cholesterol 231-255 mg % Diet contains 30% animal or solid fats	Cholesterol 256-280 mg % Diet contains 40% animal or solid fats	Cholesterol 281-300 mg % Diet contains 50% animal or solid fats
BLOOD PRESSURE	100 upper reading	120 upper reading	140 upper reading	160 upper reading	180 upper reading	200 or over upper reading
SEX	Female under 40	Female 40-50	Female over 50	Male	Stocky male	Bald stocky male

For meaningful interpretation of RISKO only the official RISKO directions should be used.

Conclusions:

1. What is your total score?

2. What is your classification?

3. What does this indicate you should do to lower your heart attack risk?

LAB 14
POSTURE ANALYSIS

NAME _____ SECTION _____ DATE _____

Posture refers to the position assumed by the body. Good posture is important for appearance, for maximal movement efficiency, to prevent soreness and muscle strains, and to enhance function of internal organs. If deviations from proper alignment are noted, it may be possible to suggest exercises to correct the problem.

Procedure

1. Have a partner assist you by comparing your alignment of various body areas with those on the Posture Rating Chart.

2. Record the score which best corresponds to your rating.

Posture Rating Chart (see next page)

Conclusions:

1. Is there a particular area of your body that seems to need improved alignment?

2. What specific exercises would be appropriate to improve your posture?

3. Do you feel you need qualified professional help to assist you?

POSTURE SCORE SHEET

					SCORING DATES		
Name							
	GOOD – 10	**FAIR – 5**	**POOR – 0**				
HEAD LEFT RIGHT	HEAD ERECT GRAVITY LINE PASSES DIRECTLY THROUGH CENTER	HEAD TWISTED OR TURNED TO ONE SIDE SLIGHTLY	HEAD TWISTED OR TURNED TO ONE SIDE MARKEDLY				
SHOULDERS LEFT RIGHT	SHOULDERS LEVEL (HORIZONTALLY)	ONE SHOULDER SLIGHTLY HIGHER THAN OTHER	ONE SHOULDER MARKEDLY HIGHER THAN OTHER				
SPINE LEFT RIGHT	SPINE STRAIGHT	SPINE SLIGHTLY CURVED LATERALLY	SPINE MARKEDLY CURVED LATERALLY				
HIPS LEFT RIGHT	HIPS LEVEL (HORIZONTALLY)	ONE HIP SLIGHTLY HIGHER	ONE HIP MARKEDLY HIGHER				
ANKLES	FEET POINTED STRAIGHT AHEAD	FEET POINTED OUT	FEET POINTED OUT MARKEDLY ANKLES SAG IN (PRONATION)				
NECK	NECK ERECT CHIN IN HEAD IN BALANCE DIRECTLY ABOVE SHOULDERS	NECK SLIGHTLY FORWARD CHIN SLIGHTLY OUT	NECK MARKEDLY FORWARD CHIN MARKEDLY OUT				
UPPER BACK	UPPER BACK NORMALLY ROUNDED	UPPER BACK SLIGHTLY MORE ROUNDED	UPPER BACK MARKEDLY ROUNDED				
TRUNK	TRUNK ERECT	TRUNK INCLINED TO REAR SLIGHTLY	TRUNK INCLINED TO REAR MARKEDLY				
ABDOMEN	ABDOMEN FLAT	ABDOMEN PROTRUDING	ABDOMEN PROTRUDING AND SAGGING				
LOWER BACK	LOWER BACK NORMALLY CURVED	LOWER BACK SLIGHTLY HOLLOW	LOWER BACK MARKEDLY HOLLOW				
			TOTAL SCORES				

Source: Reedco, Inc., Auburn, NY

LAB 15
STRESS ASSESSMENT

NAME_____ SECTION_____ DATE_____

Purpose:

1. To assist you in evaluating your current level of stress.
2. To help you assess how you are living and to alert you to some signs and sources of stress in your life.

Procedure:

Answer the following questions and score yourself accordingly.

TEST 1 — A STRESS AND TENSION TEST

	Often	Occasionally	Seldom
1. I feel tense, anxious or have nervous indigestion.	2	1	0
2. People at work/home arouse my tension.	2	1	0
3. I eat/drink/smoke in response to tension.	2	1	0
4. I have tension or migraine headaches, pain in the neck or shoulder, and insomnia.	2	1	0
5. I can't turn off my thoughts at night or on weekends to feel relaxed and refreshed for the next day.	2	1	0

	Often	Occasionally	Seldom
6. I find it difficult to concentrate on what I am doing because I am worrying about other things.	2	1	0
7. I take tranquilizers (or other drugs) to relax.	2	1	0
8. I have a difficult time finding time to relax.	2	1	0
9. Once I find the time, it is hard for me to relax.	Yes (1)	No (0)	
10. My workday is made up of too many deadlines.	Yes (1)	No (0)	

TOTAL SCORE _____

A score of 12 or higher indicates a high tension level and difficulty coping with stress in your life.

TEST 2 — SELF-ASSESSMENT

Choose the most appropriate answer for each of the following ten questions.

How often do you . . .

1. Feel stifled or held back in your personal or professional life?
   (a) almost always (b) often (c) seldom (d) almost never _____

2. Feel a need for greater accomplishment?
   (a) almost always (b) often (c) seldom (d) almost never _____

3. Feel as though your life needs guidance or direction?
   (a) almost always (b) often (c) seldom (d) almost never _____

4. Notice yourself growing impatient?
   (a) almost always (b) often (c) seldom (d) almost never   _____

5. Find yourself feeling as if you are in a "rut"?
   (a) almost always (b) often (c) seldom (d) almost never   _____

6. Find yourself disillusioned?
   (a) almost always (b) often (c) seldom (d) almost never   _____

7. Find yourself frustrated?
   (a) almost always (b) often (c) seldom (d) almost never   _____

8. Find yourself disappointed?
   (a) almost always (b) often (c) seldom (d) almost never   _____

9. Find yourself feeling inferior?
   (a) almost always (b) often (c) seldom (d) almost never   _____

10. Find yourself upset because things haven't gone according
    to plan?
    (a) almost always (b) often (c) seldom (d) almost never   _____

    Calculate your total score as follows:
    (a) = 4 Points, (b) = 3 points, (c) = 2 points, (d) = 1 point

The highest score is 40 and the lowest is 10. The higher you score, the greater your perception of frustration and the more stressful frustration will appear to you.

General Guidelines:

High frustration/high stress — 40-25
Moderate frustration/stress — 24-20
Low frustration/stress — 19-10

LAB 16
AEROBIC DANCE WORKOUT

NAME _____ SECTION _____ DATE _____

Purpose:

1. To provide you with an aerobic dance routine that you can learn and use to help you maintain your cardiovascular fitness.
2. To provide you with an outline of how to organize your workout for optimal benefits.
3. To motivate you to continue to exercise for a lifetime.

WORKOUT SCHEDULE

Frequency: Work out three to five times per week for 15 to 60 minutes depending on your fitness level and fitness goals. If you are a beginner or resuming an exercise program, begin with 3 days per week and add a day as your fitness level improves.

Intensity: Work in a range of 60 to 90% of your training heart rate range.

Warm-up: Always begin with a warm-up for approximately 8 to 10 minutes of rhythmic limbering exercises. Gradually increase the heart rate by increasing the intensity with exercises such as jogging in place. Beginners can adapt any of the following exercise to low-impact by keeping one foot on the floor at all times. Intermediate or advanced exercisers can repeat the sequences a number of times to meet the fitness goals.

Cool-down: After aerobic activity, always cool down with walking or rhythmic movements to allow the heart rate to return to its pre-existing state slowly and safely. When the heart rate is 120 beats or less, continue the cool-down with more intense stretching exercises.

The Workout: Perform each exercise for 16 repetitions to meet the minimum requirement of at least 20 minutes of aerobic activity. You can increase the intensity by raising the arms and legs higher during the

LAB 16, CONTINUED

workout. Likewise, you can decrease the intensity by doing intermittent walking in place or leg lifting. Be creative and incorporate some of your own movement ideas into your program.

After your workout, spend extra time stretching the following muscle groups, most often used during a complete aerobic workout:

1. Upper back
2. Lower back
3. Shoulders
4. Waist
5. Quadriceps (front of thigh)
6. Hamstrings (back of thigh)
7. Buttocks
8. Outer thigh, inner thigh
9. Calves

Routine # 1

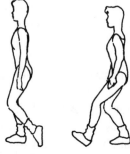

1. Toe, heel, toe, heel. Jog in place.

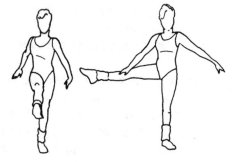

2. Step kick front, step kick side. Jog in place.

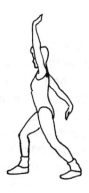

3. Pedal pusher with arms. Jog in place.

LAB 16, CONTINUED

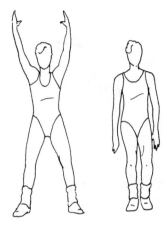

4. Jumping jacks with arms. Jog in place.

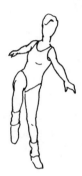

5. Skip forward and then backward. Jog in place.

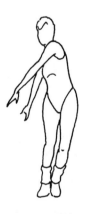

6. Twist side to side using arms. Jog in place.

7. Repeat the entire sequence.

LAB 16, CONTINUED

Routine #2

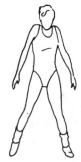

1. Begin with shoulder isolations. Run in place.

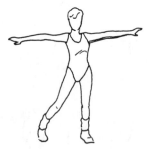

2. Slide to the right 8 counts, slide left 8 counts. Run in place.

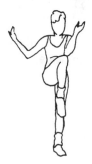

3. High leg lifting. Run in place.

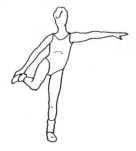

4. Heel slap. Run in place.

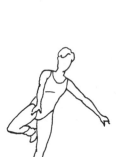

5. Step, hop, alternate right and left sides. Run in place.

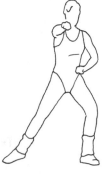

6. Side step, punch with arms. Run in place.

7. Repeat the entire sequence.

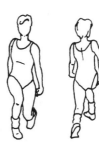

1. Begin rolling up the spine, vertebrate by vertebrate.

2. Moving forward, pivot turn and run in place. March in place.

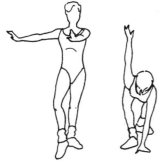

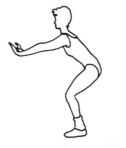

3. The Charleston (step touch front, step touch back). Jog in place.

4. Feet together, jump backwards extending the arms forward. March in place.

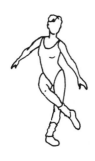

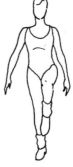

5. Polka step (heel toe, slide, slide). Run in place.

6. Schottische (run, run, run, hop). March in place. Run in place.

7. Repeat the entire sequence.

LAB 16
AEROBIC DANCE WORKOUT

NAME_____ SECTION_____ DATE_____

AEROBIC WORKOUT CHECKLIST

	Yes	No
1. Did you warm up thoroughly before beginning your routine?	____	____
2. Did you wear specifically designed aerobic shoes?	____	____
3. Did you monitor your heart rate during and after the workout?	____	____
4. Did you walk briskly and do a post-aerobic cool-down after performing your routines?	____	____
5. Did you perform appropriate cool-down exercises and stretches?	____	____
6. Did you drink fluids as necessary to replace lost body fluids?	____	____

Results:

1. Were you able to perform the dance steps and patterns in the aerobic routines? Do you think you need to improve your dance techniques?

2. Did you reach your target heart rate during the pulse check reading?

3. Do you feel you got a good workout from this program? Why or why not?

4. Will you continue to incorporate aerobic dance exercises into your fitness program? Why or why not?

INDEX